THE COMPLETE
ELDERCARE PLANNER

THE COMPLETE ELDERCARE PLANNER

*Where to Start, Questions to Ask,
and How to Find Help*

Joy Loverde

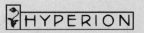

NEW YORK

An earlier edition of this book was published by
Silvercare Productions, Copyright © 1993 Joy Loverde

Revised and Updated Edition Copyright © 1997 Joy Loverde

Copyright © 1997 Joy Loverde

LIBRARY OF CONGRESS CATALOGING-IN-PUBLICATION DATA

Loverde, Joy.
The complete eldercare planner : where to start, questions to ask,
and how to find help / Joy Loverde. — 1st ed.
p.   cm.
Includes indexes.
ISBN 0-7868-8229-8
1. Aged—Home care—United States—Planning.   2. Aging parents—
Care—United States—Planning.   3. Caregivers—United States—Life
skills guides.   I. Title.
HV1461.L6843   1997
362.6—dc20   96–43370
                                                        CIP

Designed by M. J. DiMassi

FIRST EDITION
10 9 8 7 6 5 4 3 2 1

For my daughter, Bonnie Dowd

Acknowledgments

The essence of this book began when I was a student at Trinity High School in River Forest, Illinois. Something happened one cold and rainy Thanksgiving morning that would change my life forever. What I witnessed while visiting a nursing home with my classmates to cheer up elderly residents on that holiday raised questions that would haunt me throughout my adult life—*How did those elderly people end up there? What circumstances led to their hopelessness and resignation? And importantly, where were their families on this day of thanks?*

So began my life's work. I am grateful for the unflagging encouragement that I received from so many and hope to express here some fraction of my sincere thanks to those who contributed to the makings of this book.

To Bonnie Dowd and Paul Silverman, whose kindness and patience placed no limits on my writing and travel schedule and who constantly served me in love. I am grateful to them and for them.

To Alba Wright, my mother, a woman of grace who taught me how to treat elderly family members with dignity and respect through her examples of devotion while caring for her own mother, Maria Nesti.

To the Honorable Charles M. Loverde, my father, who allowed me the privilege of being his caregiver until his death.

To James, Carol, Peter, and Linda, my siblings, who travel as equal partners with me on the Loverde Family caregiving path, and in my life's actions, I hope I always show them the respect, love, and gratitude they deserve.

To Angie Thoburn and Jill Morris, two powerful and inherently wise women whose early support and validation regarding this project is simply not measurable and who leavened my life with their unconditional friendship and love.

To Jan and Scott Lane; Pat Stinson and the NESRA staff; Kathryn Cunningham; Karen

Peterson, Life Section editor of *USA Today;* Sherren Leigh and Suzanne Krill of *Today's Chicago Woman;* Beverly Kennedy, president of Kennedy and Company Public Relations; Louise Fradkin, co-founder of Children of Aging Parents, Inc.; and Beata Trudgeon for helping me to communicate the value and power of the planning approach to eldercare issues and who recognized early on my potential as the family caregiver spokesperson by inviting me to speak to a myriad of audiences.

To my dear friends and brilliant colleagues Dominic DiFrisco, senior vice-president of Burson-Marsteller, and Robert B. Blancato, executive director of the 1995 White House Conference on Aging, for their solid and steadfast feedback, encouragement, and contributions to keeping me in the aging market limelight.

To my literary agent, Joe Durepos, for his creative marketing leadership, insight, and synergistic effort in helping this book take flight. I sometimes feel he is an angel sent especially to me.

To my Hyperion editor, Lisa Jenner Hudson, for her professional competence and inner commitment to the material and for her skill and sensitivity in fulfilling that commitment. Her careful reading and many excellent suggestions have greatly improved the book from start to finish and I am most grateful to her.

And lastly, I gained incredible insight and inspiration from the late Mary Goldberg, who died at the age of 97, and Honora Bess Silverman, who shed genuine hope and light on an often dark and painful subject—aging. These women offered me the opportunity to try to understand their lives and served as role models on growing older with grace, charm, beauty, and wit, never robbing age of its great dignity and advantage.

Joy Loverde, 1997

Contents

INTRODUCTION 1

ELDER'S EMERGENCY INFORMATION 3

1. EFFECTIVE PLANNING 5

A Place to Start 5

Getting Caught Off Guard 17

Low Cost/Free Resources 21

Action Checklist 23

2. CAREGIVERS 26

How to Tell When Your Elder Needs Help 26

Share the Care 31

Take Care of You 42

Low Cost/Free Resources 46

Action Checklist 49

3. EMERGENCY PREPAREDNESS 52

Quick and Easy Access 52

Managing Medications 57

If Your Elder Is Hospitalized 64

Low Cost/Free Resources 74

Action Checklist 75

4. MONEY MATTERS 78

The Cost of Caring 78

Ready Cash 85

Low Cost/Free Resources 97

Action Checklist 100

5. LEGAL MATTERS 103

Estate Planning 103

Elder Advocacy 109

Low Cost/Free Resources 112

Action Checklist 114

6. INSURANCE 116

Insurance Coverage for a Longer Life 116

Beyond Medicare 121

Low Cost/Free Resources 127

Action Checklist 129

7. HOUSING   131

Home Suite Home   131

Low Cost/Free Resources   145

Action Checklist   148

8. SAFE AND SECURE   149

Minimize Distress over Distance   149

Low Cost/Free Resources   161

Action Checklist   163

9. TRANSPORTATION   165

Steer Clear   165

Low Cost/Free Resources   170

Action Checklist   171

10. HEALTH AND WELLNESS   172

Taking Charge: Healthy Living Tips   172

How to Communicate with the Doctor   180

Low Cost/Free Resources   189

Action Checklist   192

11. DEATH AND DYING   194

Death (and Life) Is a Matter of Attitude   194

Low Cost/Free Resources   204

Action Checklist   206

12. QUALITY OF LIFE   207

What's Age For Anyway   207

Aging with a Disability   214

Family Power   218

Low Cost/Free Resources   224

Action Checklist   227

13. DOCUMENTS LOCATOR   229

Action Checklist   249

ORGANIZATIONS INDEX   253

WEBSITE INDEX   261

SUBJECT INDEX   263

THE COMPLETE
ELDERCARE PLANNER

Introduction

What makes a person good at getting old? Perhaps the answer lies between the lines of several small-town newspaper articles I came across in my travels. One story described a seventy-three-year-old man from Iowa who completed a 240-mile trip on a riding lawn mower to visit his eighty-year-old brother in Wisconsin. He couldn't see well enough to get a driver's license but this didn't prevent him from being with his brother. Another favorite story told of a 100-year-old woman who divorced her 105-year-old husband because she said he was treating her badly and she did not want to live unhappily for the rest of her life.

The tales of these elderly people remind me of what the role of family caregiver is really about: to support the independence of our elders for as long as possible. Everyone, including the very old and the sick, has the right to decide how to live and how to die. To accept this aspect of eldercare is very difficult, especially when we do not agree or understand the choices that our aging family members make for themselves. As a result, we experience simultaneous feelings of sadness, anger, guilt, love, and helplessness. The caregiving journey leads us through unfamiliar territory and requires that we learn an entirely new set of rules and roles. We will grapple with questions like—*Who makes the decisions?* and *Who pays for what?*

For those of us who are assisting aging parents, the popular perception that at some point we become our parents' parents (commonly termed role reversal), is not true. The elderly sometimes require the kind of care and assistance typically associated with children and, at times, we may feel as though we are our parents' parents, but to treat them as such is demeaning. The common goal of family members is to become mutually responsible partners. "Partnering" with our parents is the more appropriate term when used in association with eldercare.

My approach to family caregiving is based on the principles of planning and is the secret to my effectiveness in this role. I have learned that it is better to be proactive than reactive. When I plan, I have choices; when I react my choices are limited and costly, emotionally, financially, and otherwise. Remember, perfect planning does not exist, however, *any* effort you invest in making plans with your aging relatives will have a considerable impact on the quality of your life and that of the entire family.

Aging people, in turn, present us with many gifts: the opportunity to benefit from their inherent wisdom and the privilege of assisting them in their final days. My mission is to protect and honor one of our nation's greatest resources—the elderly. I hope that you, too, find your caregiving experience rewarding and that this planner makes your journey easier along the way.

—Joy Loverde
July 10, 1995

ELDER'S EMERGENCY INFORMATION

Name _____

Address _____

City/State/Zip _____

Telephone _____

Social Security Number _____

Date of Birth _____

Blood Type _____

Allergies _____

Medications _____

Health Insurance/Policy Number _____

ELDER'S EMERGENCY TELEPHONE NUMBERS

Fire _____   Electrician _____

Police _____   Electric Co. _____

Doctor _____   Water Co. _____

Doctor _____   Gas Co. _____

Dentist _____   TV Cable Co. _____

Nurse Agency _____   Locksmith _____

Nurse _____   Plumber _____

Hospital _____   House Alarm _____

Clinic _____   Guardian _____

Pharmacy _____   Social Worker _____

Animal Hospital _____   Neighbor _____

Veterinarian _____   Neighbor _____

Auto Repair _____   Friend _____

Airline _____   Friend _____

Train _____   Friend _____

Bus _____   House Sitter _____

Spouse _____   Pet Sitter _____

Family _____   Home Care Services _____

Family _____   Lawyer _____

Family _____   Accountant _____

Family _____   Insurance Agent _____

Senior Center _____   Banker _____

Suicide Hotline _____   Co-worker _____

Clergy _____   Landlord _____

Chapter 1

EFFECTIVE PLANNING

A Place to Start

Most of us are inadequately prepared, emotionally and otherwise, to face the complex issues associated with caring for aging family members. This is because each eldercare problem can be made up of a combination of issues. How one family addresses an eldercare issue is not necessarily how another family approaches the same problem. What works one day could change drastically, overnight. How then do we proceed under these seemingly chaotic circumstances? The answer lies in planning ahead.

Planning, however, takes on a whole new level of meaning when it comes to caring for an aging relative: We family caregivers can plan on this time in our lives to be uncertain and unpredictable. Existing family decision-making patterns will no longer apply. We soon realize that we will not be returning to what we experienced as family life in our past. What we *can* plan on is a constant change in circumstances that involves the entire family—sometimes suddenly, sometimes so gradually that we may not even realize that change has occurred. No matter how carefully we make eldercare preparations, the only thing we can plan on is changing our plans.

Because the true nature of assisting an aging parent, spouse, or other family member includes a roller coaster of emotional upsets, the process of family caregiving requires nothing less than a constant management of our attitudes, choices, and plans. *The Complete Eldercare Planner* is your road map through this unfamiliar territory. Here are some suggestions for you to make the most of this book:

Read the Introduction and Objectives pages at the beginning of each chapter. Knowing what you are reading and why will be especially helpful when the emotional aspect of assisting an aging relative will undermine your ability to accomplish the eldercare task at hand.

Review each chapter, then set goals by writing them down on the Eldercare Goals Chart found on page 251. As you reach your goals, check them off on the Action Checklist at the end of each chapter. Effective planning is specific, realistic, and *written*.

Keep track of your elder's emergency telephone numbers and other important information by filling out the form on page 3 of this planner.

For fast reference on eldercare resources and websites listed throughout this planner, turn to the Index at the back of this book.

You now have the tools you need to get started.

A PLACE TO START

- Planning and preparation are critical for effective eldercare.
- Experts agree that rule number one in thoughtful planning is to use some form of planner to write things down.

Whether you are planning for future eldercare needs or helping an aging relative in a crisis situation, this planner will assist you and your family in pulling it all together.

Objectives

After completing A Place to Start you will be able to:

Create opportunities to open up the lines of communication.

Minimize the number of crisis eldercare situations.

Reduce confusion in crisis situations.

Enjoy your aging family members' later years with greater peace of mind.

PLAN ONE
Don't read this book. Use it.

This planner is specifically designed and organized to help you understand and manage issues associated with assisting an aging parent, spouse, and other relatives. *The Complete Eldercare Planner* offers immediate solutions to common problems by way of time-saving action plans, charts, and checklists. At the end of every chapter you will also find an in-depth list of nationwide resources if you need additional support.

Decide what options work best for you. How you use *The Complete Eldercare Planner* depends on the nature of your eldercare situation, your family's decision-making patterns, the help you receive from others, and the availability of financial resources. You may choose to implement one plan, several plans, or even a combination of plans. Make use of the spaces provided in this planner for notetaking, telephone numbers, goal setting, and locating documents.

Keep in mind that the process of assisting an aging relative requires assessing the situation at hand. Open up the lines of communication early with all family members and seek the advice of geriatric care professionals whenever necessary. To make assumptions about what is happening instead of talking to each other always does more harm than good. Operate from fact, not fiction.

Keep your planning and time-line expectations realistic. Ask yourself on a regular basis these three simple questions: *What can happen? What will my elder be able to do about what happens?* and *What can the rest of the family do to help?*

Plan early. The well-being of the entire family depends on the quantity and the quality of your eldercare options, decisions, and plans.

PLAN TWO
Implement planning principles.

Follow these six basic planning principles:

Set goals. Know what you are doing and why.

Create support systems and use them. Surround aging family members with people and resources to share responsibilities, exchange the rewards, and to protect against family caregiver stress.

Write it down. Put dates on all notes. Record plans, goals, ideas, phone numbers, questions, answers, promises, decisions, tasks, and appointments and keep them in a convenient, accessible location.

Organize information. Keep notes, bills, receipts, contracts, letters, brochures, and any eldercare-related information in a safe, twenty-four-hour accessible place. Create a system that makes it easy to find information when you need it.

Allow sufficient time for research. Gathering information and creating options are critical to thoughtful action. Research more than one option.

Research all costs and who pays.

PLAN THREE
Talk with your elder, not at him/her.

Make the best of every eldercare conversation with these simple reminders:

- Basic personality patterns and traits don't change; they even may become exaggerated or intensify in later years.
- Remember, eldercare discussions will come about because everyone is adapting to a loss of one kind or another.
- Keep the focus of conversations on present-day issues.
- Offer information rather than conclusions. Facilitate conversations in terms of questions, not answers.
- Ease into conversations. The more informal and relaxed the better.
- Present one idea at a time.
- Allow time for everyone to adjust and react to discussions.
- Never do for your elders what they can do for themselves.

PLAN FOUR
Be prepared for the runaround.

Gathering information, locating resources, and getting eldercare services in motion can cause a great deal of anxiety. Detailed application processes, waiting lists, lengthy interviews, document searching, being put on hold, outdated telephone numbers, and other stressful situations are common. Use this planner to guide you through the eldercare maze.

Make telephone calls and attend appointments with paper and pen in hand. Confirm in-person appointments a day in advance. Arrange to have someone accompany your elder to *every* appointment. Distribute copies of documents while keeping the originals for yourself. Evaluate the quality of services you and your family members receive and report anyone who treats you disrespectfully.

Ask the following questions where applicable and keep a written record of the answers:

What is your name and your title?
Are you a staff member or a volunteer?
How much do services cost?
What is the average cost for my particular needs?
Are fees or commissions negotiable? Sliding scale?
Are initial consultations available free of charge?
What other costs should I anticipate?
Are payment plans available?
Does insurance cover costs?
Are costs tax deductible?
Will you assign someone to assist me?
What documents are needed? Originals? Copies?
Will you put fees/estimates in writing?
Will you itemize bills?
Do you have brochures/literature you can send me?
Will you provide references? credentials?
Will you provide written contracts? regulations?
Are you a member of any professional organization?
Are you certified? Licensed? Bonded?
What free services are available?
Will you put me on your mailing list?
Do you provide pickup and delivery service? Transportation?
Can your office accommodate a wheelchair?
Do you have telecommunication access for hearing or visually impaired?
Are home visits available?
Are you located near public transportation?

What days/hours are you open for business?
Is there an emergency number when the office is closed?

PLAN FIVE
List and prioritize your eldercare concerns.

Refer to this planner's Contents for a review of eldercare issues. Prioritize which issues must be dealt with immediately. Consider both long-term and short-term options.

Given the opportunity, most aging people would choose to stay in their own homes. As the aging population grows, so, too, are the number of assisted-living options that allow them to do so. Assessing and arranging for eldercare services, however, is a complex experience. This is because:

- Every aging person requires a unique combination of eldercare services.
- Each community and state offers a variety of eldercare programs listed under different names.
- All the eldercare services are rarely available from one source.
- The eligibility process for public programs is complicated.

PLAN SIX
Make good use of the local and national eldercare resources listed throughout this planner.

The eldercare service providers and organizations listed at the end of every chapter assist family members in many ways. If you are unsure of the services your relative needs or are searching for a specific service provider, use the lists below as a quick guide to find what you are looking for.

Whether you are providing family caregiving assistance from the next community or the next state, also obtain copies of your elder's community telephone directories—the white and yellow pages. Update these directories yearly.

Look under the following headings in the yellow pages to get the telephone numbers of these eldercare resources where your aging family member resides:

- Hospital *(Ask for the discharge planner.)*
- Social Service Organizations

- Religious Congregations
- Senior Centers

Look under the following headings in the blue pages to obtain the telephone numbers of these government offices:

- Area agency on aging
- Department of Insurance *(Medicare)*
- Department of Mental Health and Developmental Disabilities
- Department of Public Aid *(food stamps, Medicaid)*
- Department of Public Health
- Department of Rehabilitation Services
- Department of Revenue *(tax relief)*
- Department of Transportation *(reduced fares, taxi coupons)*
- Department of Veterans' Benefits

Call the local hospital, social service organizations, religious congregations, and senior centers to obtain information regarding:

- Free brochures and community eldercare directories
- Books, tapes, videos on eldercare-related topics
- Caregiver newsletters
- On-line computer services
- Physician referrals
- Community education programs
- Prerecorded health information
- Registered nurse telephone advice
- Infusion services
- Hospice
- Behavioral health programs
- Home respiratory services
- Nursing and personal care
- Chronic disease management
- Home medical equipment
- Hotline telephone numbers
- Caregiver support groups
- Parish nurse services
- Volunteer programs

- Benefits eligibility
- Community health fairs
- International eldercare resources
- Foreign language services

Use the following lists to get recommendations on specific eldercare services in your elder's hometown.

Homemaker Services *(house cleaning, personal care, errands, cooking):*
- Area agency on aging
- Church groups
- Civic groups
- Social services organizations
- Visiting Nurses Association
- The Red Cross
- Home care agency
- Family and friend referrals
- Classified newspaper ads

Home Repair/Maintenance Services *(upkeep, installations, improvements):*
- Area agency on aging
- Social services organizations
- Neighborhood improvement programs
- Church groups

Nutrition Sites/Meals Programs *(home delivered meals, group meals):*
- Area agency on aging
- Church groups
- Senior centers
- Hospital discharge planner

Companion Services *(friendly visits to homebound elderly):*
- Area agency on aging
- Church groups
- Hospital discharge planner
- Neighborhood clubs
- Social services organizations
- Civic groups

- Volunteer organizations
- YMCA/YWCA
- City recreation department
- Hospice volunteers
- Youth groups

Telephone Reassurance *(daily contact for aging people who live alone):*
- Police department
- Hospital discharge planner
- Senior centers
- Social services organizations
- Civic groups
- Home health-care agency

Observation Programs *(Letter carriers and utility workers are trained to identify signs that an elderly person may need help.):*
- Public utility office
- Post office
- Area agency on aging
- Community-watch program

Transportation Services *(Van services are available to disabled elderly people who need to attend medical appointments.):*
- Area agency on aging
- Home health-care agency
- Hospital discharge planner
- Public health department
- Social services organizations
- Church groups
- Civic groups
- The Red Cross

Housing Options *(from retirement communities to skilled nursing care):*
- Retirement communities
- Area agency on aging
- State ombudsman office
- Senior centers
- Hospital discharge planner

Home Health-Care Services *(from managing medications to skilled nursing care):*
- Visiting Nurses Association
- Area agency on aging
- Social services organizations
- Home health-care agency
- Public department of family services
- Hospital discharge planner
- United Way

Hospice Programs *(care and counseling for dying patients and their family members):*
- Hospital discharge planner
- American Cancer Society
- Visiting Nurses Association
- Church groups
- Social services organizations

Emergency Response Systems *(transmitters to call for help):*
- Hospital discharge planner
- Fire Department

Respite Care Services *(providing time off for family caregivers):*
- Hospital discharge planner
- Nursing homes
- Senior centers
- Social services organizations
- Home health-care agency
- State ombudsman office

PLAN SEVEN
Have a plan to accomplish eldercare goals if the lines of communication go down.

Creating backup plans must be your prime consideration if and when your aging family member does not want to discuss eldercare issues with you. Review the action plan suggestions in each chapter of this planner to be well informed of your options.

In the meantime, it may be possible for others to keep the lines of communication open. Enlist the help of family members, clergy, family doctor, lawyer, accountant, friends, neighbors, and co-workers.

Getting Caught Off Guard

The responsibilities associated with eldercare are often initiated in a crisis and can catch us by surprise whether we anticipate them or not. This section of the planner offers family members proven, effective methods of handling eldercare problems when important caregiving conversations and decisions did not take place ahead of time. It is specifically designed to guide you through the caregiving process in the absence of planning.

The advent of an eldercare crisis typically brings strong, sometimes opposing emotions to the surface. Love and anger, in particular, seem to go hand-in-hand. These feelings can be so intense that they may temporarily immobilize family caregivers. This is normal. The first course of action in the event of an unexpected eldercare problem is to accept the circumstance as is and focus on creating solutions that address the needs of the entire family.

To gain an understanding of the problem, to research options, to be resourceful, to communicate responsibly, and to seek assistance are your immediate goals and the keys to surviving this confusing ordeal. Don't let anyone rush you. Resist the temptation to make quick decisions. Take it one step at a time. You are in more control of the situation than you think.

GETTING CAUGHT OFF GUARD

- Our lives are changing at a faster rate than at any other time in human history. Sometimes we can plan for change, other times we are caught completely off guard.
- Addressing unexpected eldercare problems step-by-step builds a caregiver's skills and confidence in mastering change.
- When it comes to caring for aging relatives, there is no such thing as staying in control. The best we can do is to build and maintain positive attitudes toward change.

In the absence of planning, family caregivers can implement proven strategies that help them handle eldercare situations effectively.

Objectives

After completing Getting Caught Off Guard you will be able to:

Compile eldercare planning tools.

Accumulate eldercare resources.

Maintain an informal network of support.

Access eldercare expert advice.

Create opportunities to make informed decisions.

PLAN ONE
Plan for action.

In the absence of eldercare plans and discussions, follow these tips to get you pointed in the right direction:

Get organized. *The Complete Eldercare Planner* offers family members immediate assistance. Turn to this planner's Contents to determine which eldercare topic needs attention today. Follow that chapter's action plans and checklists. Next, complete The Documents Locator section of the planner as soon and as much as possible. Create a file on each aging family member and store the information in one convenient, twenty-four-hour accessible location. Have access to a copy machine, facsimile (fax) service, and overnight mail service.

Write everything down. Date your notes. Record conversations (in-person and on telephone), names, addresses, telephone numbers, options, decisions, ideas, questions, answers, plans, promises, instructions, directions—everything.

Obtain copies of telephone directories. Have access to your elder's community telephone books (white and yellow pages) and personal address book.

Create a helper's list. Make a list of people who can help you including other family members, friends and neighbors, co-workers, church members, support groups, and volunteers. Record their home and work telephone numbers. Make copies of this list and distribute to family and friends. Keep a copy at home and at work. Call or write to the low cost/free resource organizations listed at the end of each chapter if you need additional assistance.

Make lists. Keep track of day-to-day caregiving tasks like errands, cooking, housekeeping, and shopping. When people ask how they can help, let them choose from your list. If they don't ask, pick up the telephone and solicit their assistance. The reality is, you're going to need help with eldercare responsibilities whether you realize it or not.

Access eldercare professionals. Obtain the telephone numbers of those professionals who assist your aging relative like doctors, dentist, hospital staff, pharmacist, police, insurance agents, lawyer, accountant, and clergy.

PLAN TWO
Seek expert advice.

Professional eldercare advice, referrals, and assistance are a telephone call away. Contact the local hospital and ask for the **discharge planner**. You also can call the local chapter of the **Visiting Nurses Association** and the local **department on aging** for information regarding home health-care services and to gain access to even more community resources and service providers.

If your aging family member lives out of town you can employ the services of a **geriatric case manager**. These experts will make an on-site visit to your relative, assess the situation at hand, then make any necessary care arrangements. Be prepared for steep hourly rates—from $50 to $175 an hour plus an assessment fee. However, hiring these geriatric professionals for several hours may well be worth the price, especially in an eldercare emergency. Call the hospital discharge planner for referrals.

PLAN THREE
Make informed decisions.

Keep family members informed and involved for effective results:

- Ask questions of all health care and service providers until you are completely satisfied that you have explored all options.
- Allow sufficient time for research for the purpose of making thoughtful, informed decisions.
- Research all costs and who pays.
- Check all references.
- Get legal advice on anything that requires contracts and money deposits.
- Insist on continuous family discussions. Keep everyone involved and responsible.
- Make sure your aging family members are involved in their own decision-making process.

Low Cost/Free Resources

The **telephone directory** is a major source of information. The front section of this directory includes resources for Community Access, Emergency Preparedness, and Government Agencies. The yellow pages will be useful to locate service providers. Also get a copy of your elder's community telephone books. Update these directories yearly.

Call the **area agency on aging** for community programs assisting the elderly. The phone number is listed in the blue pages of the telephone directory.

AARP (American Association of Retired Persons) is a powerful organization assisting the elderly. Look them up in the white pages of the telephone directory.

Hospital discharge planners can provide current information and referrals on local eldercare services. Also inquire about a community eldercare resource directory, which is usually free for the asking.

The **public library** is stocked with books on related subjects. Get to know the experts at the reference desk.

Local newspapers and radio and television stations often advertise **free community programs** conducted by eldercare experts, health care providers, financial and legal advisors, and members of local social and business organizations.

Rent **videos** on related subjects.

Research **on-line computer websites.**

Call the **mayor's office** to get the information or help you need.

Masonic Orders, Rotary Clubs, Lions Clubs, Odd Fellows Lodges, veterans' organizations, unions, business clubs, and teachers' associations provide special services to members and nonmembers alike. Refer to the yellow pages under **Associations.**

Almost all religious groups provide volunteer services for their members. Refer to **Religious Organizations** in the yellow pages.

Public and private schools, universities, and trade schools are a valuable source of information, resources, and referrals. See **Schools** in the yellow pages. Ask for the adult education and community services programs.

Local **Community Action Commissions (CAC)** and **family service agencies** offer services for low-income, minority, frail, and homebound persons including social, educational, and recreational activities.

Community **Senior Centers** provide a variety of services and activities to elderly persons including recreation, social gatherings, meals, transportation, and education.

ORGANIZATIONS

Administration on Aging's Directory of Web Aging Sites
Website *http://www.aoa.dhhs.gov/aoa/webres/craig.htm*

American Association of Retired Persons (AARP)
Fulfillment, 601 E St., NW, Washington, DC 20049, (202) 434-2277,
(800) 424-3410
Website *http://www.aarp.org*

Center for the Study of Aging
1331 H St., NW, Suite 110, Washington, DC 20005, (202) 737-4650,
(800) 221-4272

Eldercare Web
Website *http://www.ice.net/stevens/elderweb.htm*

National Association of Area Agencies on Aging
1112 16th St., NW, Suite 100, Washington, DC 20036, (202) 296-8130

National Council on the Aging, Inc.
409 Third St., SW, Second Floor, Washington, DC 20024, (202) 479-1200,
(800) 424-9046

Senior Options
Website *http://senioroptions.com*

Action Checklist

A PLACE TO START	To Do By	Completed
Set planning goals . . .		
short-term	_____	❏
long-term	_____	❏
Create a system for recording, duplicating, and filing . . .		
eldercare information	_____	❏
notes	_____	❏
questions	_____	❏
goals	_____	❏
lists	_____	❏
documents	_____	❏
phone numbers	_____	❏
agreements	_____	❏
Have access to . . .		
telephone	_____	❏
transportation	_____	❏
copy machine	_____	❏
facsimile	_____	❏
post office	_____	❏
public library	_____	❏
Review effective communication techniques (Plan Three).	_____	❏
List and prioritize eldercare concerns(Plan Five) . . .		
short-term	_____	❏
long-term	_____	❏
Contact eldercare resources (Plan Six).	_____	❏
Create a backup plan (Plan Seven).	_____	❏
Attend community eldercare programs.	_____	❏

GETTING CAUGHT OFF GUARD	To Do By	Completed

Get organized (Plan One) ...

review Table of Contents	_____	❑
prioritize issues	_____	❑
create file on elder	_____	❑
complete Documents Locator	_____	❑
store information in safe place	_____	❑

Take notes (Plan One) ...

names and addresses	_____	❑
telephone numbers	_____	❑
plans	_____	❑
instructions	_____	❑
directions	_____	❑
decisions	_____	❑
promises	_____	❑

Get telephone books ...

white pages	_____	❑
yellow pages	_____	❑
elder's white pages	_____	❑
elder's yellow pages	_____	❑

Create helper's list (Plan One) ...

family	_____	❑
friends	_____	❑
neighbors	_____	❑
co-workers	_____	❑
church members	_____	❑
volunteers	_____	❑

Copy and distribute help list to key persons (Plan One).   _____   ❑

Make list of help needed (Plan One).   _____   ❑

Ask and accept help (Plan One).   _____   ❑

Create list of eldercare advisors (Plan One).   _____   ❑

Access eldercare experts (Plan Two) . . .

hospital discharge planner	_____	❏
Visiting Nurses Association	_____	❏
local department on aging	_____	❏
geriatric case manager	_____	❏

Make informed decisions (Plan Three) . . .

questions answered to satisfaction	_____	❏
time allowed for research	_____	❏
costs investigated	_____	❏
references checked	_____	❏
legal counsel sought for contracts	_____	❏
family discussions ongoing	_____	❏
elder involved in decisions	_____	❏

Chapter 2

CAREGIVERS

How to Tell When Your Elder Needs Help

Contrary to the way elderly people are typically portrayed in advertisements and movies, getting old does not mean being helpless or losing one's memory. Unnecessary problems in the caregiving process develop when we equate aging with decline and pathology. Eldercare is defined by ability, not age. Inappropriate and inaccurate media messages of incompetence and dementia are so convincing that even our elders sometimes believe the stereotypes are true.

Aging people are people in transition. The loss of family members and friends, a change in living arrangements, the repositioning of finances, retirement, the loss of driving privileges, even the death of a pet are lifestyle transitions that require the entire family's attention. Ideally, our elders will ask for our help during times like these—but, as family members have learned, this may not happen. In fact, one aging parent might "cover up" for the other, or an aging spouse may decline assistance from the other because he/she feels ashamed and powerless.

Remember, most elderly people wish to remain independent and in control of their own lives for as long as possible. This section of the planner suggests ways that caregivers can help their aging family members remain independent by making astute observations, asking revealing questions, and paying attention to telltale signs that indicate your elder may need assistance now.

HOW TO TELL WHEN YOUR ELDER NEEDS HELP

- Adult children and spouses need not anticipate the time to intervene in the lives of their aging family members. Ideally their elders will accept lifestyle changes and request assistance.
- One aging spouse may "cover up" for the other, and problems may go undetected for years.
- Sometimes changes in mental ability, energy level, and lack of mobility are so gradual that family members may adapt to such circumstances without acknowledging that problems exist.

If you suspect that your aging relative is losing the ability to perform basic tasks, pay attention to telltale signs that indicate he/she needs immediate attention.

Objectives

After completing How to Tell When Your Elder Needs Help you will be able to:

Detect eldercare situations that require immediate attention.

Enlist your elder's help with recognizing lifestyle changes.

Prevent caregiver overinvolvement with eldercare issues.

Employ effective communication techniques.

PLAN ONE
Know what to look for.

Things may seem normal on the outside. Some changes are barely noticeable. Once in a while we all forget details or put things off—but when a *pattern* of neglect develops, it may be serious. Remember, dementia (mental deterioration) is *not* a normal part of aging. Make astute observations and recognize patterns of consistent neglect with the following:

Basic tasks—difficulty walking, dressing, talking, eating, cooking, step climbing, managing medications.

Hygiene—infrequent bathing, unusually sloppy appearance, foul mouth odor.

Responsibilities—mail unopened, papers piling up, checkbook unreadable, bills unpaid, bank account overdraft notices present, prescriptions unfilled, phone calls not returned, dirty dishes piled in sink, pots look like they have been burned, refrigerator stinks when opened, food supply is low, houseplants not watered, home interior or exterior unkempt, bathroom tile is moldy, laundry piling up, fire hazards present, new automobile dents.

Health—weight loss, loss of appetite, unhealthy eating habits, problems swallowing, lack of exercise, no energy, skin burns, black and blue marks (may be signs of falling), hearing loss (look for signs of lip reading and talking loudly), seems withdrawn without reason, bed wetting (urinary incontinence), spilling and dropping things (check carpet for stains), complains of muscle weakness, insomnia or excess sleeping, complains of dehydration (thirsty).

Isolation—not maintaining outside friendships or interests, no hobbies, phone doesn't ring, curtains drawn day and night, no transportation available, lives in another city or state and lives alone.

Attitude—cries frequently, verbally or physically abusive, talks about being depressed, abusing alcohol or drugs, less ambition and interest in fewer and fewer things, paranoid, refuses to communicate, extremely argumentative, has undergone a recent emotional or medical crisis.

Cognitive functions—consistent memory lapses, confusion, loss of reasoning skills, difficulty answering questions, gets lost walking or driving, inability to find the right word, repetitive, wears same clothes over and over, severe personality changes, wanders, cannot recall names of familiar people or objects, unable to complete a sentence, no sense of time.

Expect the unexpected. This attitude will help you to proactively detect problems and make a big difference in creating eldercare options and solutions.

PLAN TWO
Encourage your elder to take responsibility for necessary life changes.

When eldercare issues demand attention, family caregivers should keep aging relatives involved in their own decision-making process. This fosters mutually responsible partnerships between family members. Enlist your elder in recognizing that a problem exists.

Ask revealing questions (in person and on the telephone) such as . . .

Is something bothering you?
Is there something you would like to talk about?
I see (hear) that you're upset. Would you like to talk about it?
I can see (hear) that this is very important to you.

Then offer limited assistance with questions such as . . .

What can you do about this problem?
What have you done so far to solve the problem?
What are your options?
What else can you do?
Given what you already know, what do you think is your next step?
Where can you get more information?
Who can help you with this?

Give your full attention when your relative responds. Silence is a powerful communication tool. If you are perceived as a good listener, family members will be encouraged to give you important information and may be more willing later on to compromise during difficult situations.

If the answers seem impractical, ask further questions that lead to your elder's own ability to conclude whether or not his/her response is realistic:

How do you plan to accomplish what you want?
If your plan doesn't work, what else will you do?

Despite your good intentions, aging family members may not welcome any inquiries regarding existing or future eldercare issues. When this happens, remove yourself from the situation and call upon the assistance of someone else who has more influence in talking with your elder—another family member, your elder's friends and neighbors, the family doctor, or a member of the clergy may be more effective during these times.

Share the Care

The American family has undergone big changes. Medical breakthroughs mean people are living longer. For the first time in history, families have more parents than kids. Nobody's home anymore. We spend the majority of our time at work, at school, at play. We have created artificial families; hospitals, schools, churches, and companies have replaced home. There is more physical distance between families; caregivers and aging family members live an average of 100 miles away from each other.

Because of these modern realities, an important goal of this section of the planner is to expand your definition of care. Too often, family caregivers have a rigid concept of care and make statements like, "My mother will never go to a nursing home." For other caregivers it is a point of pride not to ask for help. These kinds of attitudes are unhealthy.

When we come face-to-face with our own limits and can't provide the care we wish we could, we feel it's our own fault. The truth is that we may not be the most qualified person to take on certain caregiving responsibilities. Limitations of relationships, time, stamina, and skill dictate how much help we can realistically offer.

SHARE THE CARE

- You and you alone cannot assist your elder.
- Limitations of time, stamina, and skill can make you realize that there is just so much you can do, especially if you are providing care from a distance.
- Dealing with aging family members from a distance may be the same as dealing with strangers—there can be so much you do not know.

One of the most important tasks in helping your elder is finding and creating a support network—family, friends, and professionals.

Objectives

After completing Share the Care you will be able to:

Create a network of professionals and resources to assist you.

Consider cost-effective eldercare options.

Spend more time pursuing your own personal and professional interests.

Plan One
Make a list of the tasks you can do and the ones you can't do or don't want to do.

If you are assisting an aging relative who is experiencing health care problems, ask the doctor to explain the levels of care your elder will require now and in the future. If your parent, spouse, or other relatives are caring for another aging family member, acknowledge the load they are carrying and offer to help whenever you can. Following are some of the caregiving tasks you may have to address:

Homemaker services—household maintenance, repairs, housekeeping, cleaning, laundry, errands, grocery shopping, cooking, transportation, paying bills, interacting with eldercare advisors.

Personal care—bathing, dressing, feeding, toileting, shaving, grooming, bed and chair transferring.

Home health care—skilled nursing care, hospice, managing medications, patient instruction, physical therapy, nutrition counseling.

Quality of life—companionship, escort, checking in, social activities, exercise, counseling, civic involvement, reading, religious activities, senior advocacy.

Plan Two
Identify caregivers and tasks.

The help that we caregivers receive from our informal network of support may be more readily available, reliable, and affordable than paid care providers. Create a list of people who can help you and your elder. Write down their names, addresses, home and work telephone numbers and be upfront with them about being reached twenty-four hours a day, seven days a week:

Mother	Elder's neighbors
Father	In-laws
Siblings	Children
Spouse	Nephews
Elder's friends	Nieces

Uncles	Cousins
Aunts	Co-workers
Neighbors	Stepchildren
Clergy	Grandchildren

Distribute copies of this list to your elder, siblings, relatives, spouse, children, friends, and a trusted co-worker. Keep copies in several convenient locations: near the telephone, on the refrigerator, at work, in the glove compartment of your car.

Now that you know who can help you, define how they help. Make a list of the kind of services that are needed. The next time someone says, "What can I do?" let them pick from your list. Update this list regularly since your needs and the needs of your aging family members will certainly change.

It is true that the responsibilities of eldercare within the family may be unevenly and perhaps unfairly distributed. To address this, get in the habit of speaking to other family members about your elder on a regular basis. Compare notes and try to listen with an open mind. If any family member seems reluctant to help, ask that person to contribute financially as a way to be of assistance; then you decide how to make the best use of the money.

PLAN THREE
Identify a professional network of paid care providers.

Specialized care providers can make home care a solution to institutionalized care. If you are unsure of what kind of help is needed, or where it will come from, or what it will cost, or what entitlement programs are available, you might want to hire a **geriatric case manager.** Case managers are highly trained social workers and nurses who have experience working with older adults. Case management services, however, are not usually covered by insurance. Call the hospital discharge planner for referrals.

To find reliable, competent in-home helpers, ask people you know like family, friends, and co-workers who have had successful dealings with service providers. Also ask the doctor, licensed homemaker and home-care agencies, home health care agencies, the area agency on aging, the hospital discharge planner, social service agencies, licensed nurse agencies, social workers, clergy, and an employment agency.

Another resource is the "situations wanted" column in the classified ads if you are looking to hire someone who does home care on a private basis and is self-employed. Independent workers tend to have more flexible schedules and charge less than an agency.

If none of these leads prove successful, put an ad in the paper. Rent a post box and request resumes and references.

PLAN FOUR
Be prepared with specific questions when hiring in-home helpers.

Before beginning the interview process, think about what services you need from the helper. When a job applicant calls, give a short job description, time and day expectations, salary, and benefits. Grant interviews only to those considered for the position. Arrange for other family members or a friend to be present during interviews for feedback and support. *Check all references before hiring.* Consider requesting a police report.

Ask applicant . . .

What makes you interested in this kind of work?
Tell me about your past home-care work experience.
Why did you leave your last position?
Have you received any special training?
Do you have any problems that might hinder you in this job?
How do you feel about alcohol, drugs, smoking?
Do you like cats? Dogs?
Is there anything about this job that you would not be willing to do?
What is your time commitment to this position?
Are you willing to do household chores like cooking and light housekeeping?
How flexible is your schedule?
Do you have a current driver's license?
Do you have a car available? Can you drive my car? Do you have car insurance?
What would you do if you are ill and cannot come to work?
What would you do in the case of an emergency?

Ask agency . . .

Are you licensed and accredited? By whom?
Is your agency bonded? Is your worker bonded?
Who pays insurance, taxes, and handles employer responsibilities?
How long have you been in business?
Do you accept Medicare?

Do you offer sliding-scale fees?

What are the fees for services provided by your worker?

What costs are not covered?

Who pays the worker, you or I?

What are the minimum and maximum hours of service?

Are there limits to services provided?

What is your screening process when hiring workers?

How do you supervise your workers?

Is the worker specially trained to work with older adults?

Do you find a replacement if your worker is ill or on vacation?

Do I continue to pay your worker while my relative is in the hospital?

Can your agency provide me with references on you and your worker?

What is the procedure when a worker does not show up?

How soon can a worker begin?

Ask reference . . .

How long have you known this applicant?

What was the applicant's position and job description?

How well did applicant get along with others?

What were applicant's strengths? Weaknesses?

Did you find applicant trustworthy?

Were you aware of any substance abuse? Smoking?

Would you rehire applicant?

Why did applicant leave?

Describe job, then ask if applicant is well-suited for the job.

Ask yourself . . .

Do I really believe this person is right for the job?

Will this person take charge and quickly respond in an emergency?

Is this person organized? Neat? Flexible? Energetic? Pleasant?

Does this person have the training and experience for this job?

Will this person get along with my elder? Family? Others?

Will this person know when to consult the family?

Will this person be sensitive to family traditions?

Do family members like and trust this person?

Do family members believe this person can handle this job?

PLAN FIVE
Develop a job contract for paid care providers.

Clarify duties with a formalized agreement. Modify the contract as needed. Have your employee sign a contract *before* work begins. Include the following information in the agreement:

- Employer name, address, telephone number
- Employee name, address, telephone number
- Employee Social Security number
- Salary, payment method, terms of payment *(weekly, bimonthly)*
- Benefits *(meals, entertainment allowance, vacation, insurance)*
- Expenses, transportation fees, reimbursement procedures
- Record keeping/Taxes
- Work schedule/Time keeping
- Length of service
- Illness/Absences
- Holidays/Makeup time
- Job description
- Emergency procedures
- Worker's emergency contacts *(names, day and evening telephone numbers)*
- House rules *(smoking, drinking, foul language, tardiness, absence without notice, guests)*
- Termination of employment *(two weeks, two warnings)*
- Reasons for termination *(theft, carelessness, failure to carry out duties, breaking house rules, physical or verbal abuse)*
- Quitting job procedure
- Employee signature and date
- Employer signature and date

PLAN SIX
Take steps to assure quality service from care providers.

Financial and legal considerations—Social Security contributions (FICA), federal unemployment tax (FUTA), state unemployment tax, and state workmen's compensation contributions—are the responsibility of employers when hiring paid care providers. Review employment regulations by contacting the Social Security office or the IRS office. Getting advice from an accountant or lawyer will also be helpful. Keep careful records. Notify your insurance agent about proper coverage while employing someone in the home.

The salary range for services begins at minimum wage and depends on the amount of training and experience the worker has and whether or not an agency is involved. Transportation fees may be extra. Medicare, private health insurance, and health maintenance organizations apply restrictions on home-care coverage.

Hiring a worker from an agency or business does not guarantee the quality of services provided. In fact, many new eldercare services have become available but do not have government regulation or certification programs. The state long-term care ombudsman and the area agency on aging are reliable resources for doing a background check on care providers.

It is important for family members to continuously monitor the quantity and quality of services rendered. Follow these suggestions:

- Make regular contact with your relative's care providers—by phone, mail, and better yet, in person. Exchange telephone numbers and let them know they can call you collect if they need you.
- Hire workers from agencies that are licensed, insured, and bonded. Unfortunate incidents with helpers include physical and verbal abuse and stealing.
- Write down and discuss all special instructions. Demonstrate tasks if necessary.
- Provide the care providers with emergency telephone numbers. Post this information near a telephone. Have the care providers give you the names and telephone numbers of their emergency contacts and health insurance carrier.
- Keep the care providers updated on your relative's health condition and in turn, have them contact you if they notice any changes.
- Be on the lookout for signs of trouble: The day's work is not done; The worker does not keep track of spending money; Your relative complains about the worker's attitude and quality of care; Clothes, food, and household items are missing; The worker comes late and leaves early; You feel as though you are not getting important information. Do not let problems build up. Take the time to discuss and resolve issues as they occur.
- Be aware that if the care provider is from a different cultural background, communication styles will vary from yours. For instance, asking personal questions and saying no to an authority figure may not be acceptable behavior.

• Provide encouragement and support. Let them know you appreciate their assistance. Thank you notes, flowers, and satisfied reports can really make a difference and may cause that person to pay even closer attention to your relative's well-being.

PLAN SEVEN
Take formal action if you are dissatisfied with the quality of care.

Many hospitals in the United States have a **patient representative** on staff. This advocate guides the patient through the medical bureaucracy and ensures the patient of getting the rights to which he/she is entitled, including respectful care, treatment options, and confidentiality.

An **ombudsman** monitors nursing and board and care facilities. Call this advocate if your family member is ill-treated. The ombudsman will investigate and refer the case to the state licensing agent. Refer to the telephone directory white pages under long-term-care ombudsman.

Complaints about long-term care facilities and residential care facilities can be directed to the **state department of social services,** the **state department of health services** and the **county licensing offices.** Licensing and certification reports are public information.

PLAN EIGHT
Bridge the gap in eldercare by using community programs.

Making use of community programs helps to keep aging people independent and in contact with others who can monitor their health and safety. Programs include:

Home-delivered meals—(Also known as **mobile wheels** or **meals-on-wheels**) Meals delivered to the home help homebound elders to eat right and provide an opportunity to interact with the volunteers who bring the food.

Emergency response devices—Your elderly relative wears a bracelet or necklace equipped with a radio transmitter that is activated by pushing a button. A message is sent to the hospital, police, or an emergency contact. Other programs require your family member to check in by telephone on a daily basis. When no contact is made, a designated person checks on your elder.

Carrier alert—(Also known as **postal alert**) A mail carrier who notices an unusual accumulation of mail will alert a postal supervisor to designate a person to check on your elder.

Social day care—These community programs provide several hours a day of social interaction, recreation, group meals, and supervision for aging people who cannot be safely left home alone.

Adult day health care—Supervised day care for adults is a more specialized kind of program than social day care and may include comprehensive services ranging from health assessment and nursing care to social and recreational activities. To participate in these programs usually requires a physician's prescription. Adult day health care centers are not necessarily federally licensed. To evaluate a facility . . .

- Request a *written* target enrollment policy statement.
- Ask about their policy to include patients who are actively abusing alcohol or drugs.
- Ask if facility requests updates on patient's medical records.
- Find out how the facility provides reports on the patient's activities.
- Review the staff/patient ratio. One staff member to every eight patients is typical. In cases where patients are severely mentally and physically impaired, one staff member to every five patients is an acceptable ratio.
- Ask if staff members include a director with a professional degree in the field of health and human services, a social worker, a registered nurse or licensed practical nurse supervised by an R.N.

Respite care—The time when someone takes over the care of an aging relative in order to give family caregivers relief. Respite care can be for several hours, one day, a weekend, or even a month and is available in or outside the home. Take advantage of the benefits respite care has to offer when you are unsure of decisions regarding your relative's permanent living arrangements. Optional respite care facilities outside the home include hospitals and nursing homes.

To get referrals for these community programs, call the area agency on aging, the social service agency, the family service agency, the hospital discharge planner, nursing homes, the Visiting Nurses Association, and the post office. Look in the yellow pages under Nurse and Nurse Registries, Home Health Agencies, Senior Services Organizations, and Adult Day Care Centers.

PLAN NINE
Identify volunteer resources.

Volunteers are available to assist family caregivers. Call these resources to find out what they have to offer:

Community centers	Seniors' organizations	Advocacy leagues
Senior centers	Religious organizations	Recreation centers
Hospitals	Health care providers	Grade school
Hospice	Fraternal orders	High school
Public library	Homeowners' associations	Community colleges
Aging agencies	Youth clubs	University
Family service agencies	Women's organizations	Transportation agencies
Support groups	Neighborhood groups	Veterans' organizations
Nursing agencies	Business associations	Financial institutions
Charities	Retirement organizations	Legal institutions
Church groups	Volunteer organizations	Department stores

Take Care of You

Planning ahead certainly will help family members avoid an eldercare crisis, but remember, our attitudes will greatly affect what happens when we assist aging relatives. Feelings of guilt often override other emotions and, as a result, we may be reluctant to delegate eldercare tasks. Moreover, we may feel as though we are neglecting our responsibilities by allowing someone else to relieve us, even for a short time.

Your own health, the quality of your professional and personal life, and your relationships outside of the one you have with your elder need not suffer as a consequence of providing eldercare. Ask and accept help from others, even when you are able and available to perform caregiving tasks. Make ongoing requests of assistance from other family members, friends, community resources, and volunteers. Get others used to the idea that you need their help.

You and your elder need breathing room. You may need a break from caregiving responsibilities and he/she may need a break from you. If your aging family member resents having someone else take your place temporarily, resist the temptation to cancel your plans. This section of the planner will show you how to maintain a life of your own.

TAKE CARE OF YOU

- According to Children of Aging Parents, Inc., family members provide 80 percent of the care of aging relatives. They do so without pay, often with little or no assistance, and while coping with competing responsibilities of family, work, and personal interests.
- When an aging family member lives at a distance, you may experience an overwhelming sense of helplessness.
- Family caregiving can be rewarding. But a caregiver who does not ask or accept help from others can become frustrated, develop feelings of isolation, and experience anger toward their elder and other family members.

Everyone may become a family caregiver at some time. Take steps to minimize the pressures.

Objectives

*After completing **Take Care of You** you will be able to:*

Recognize the emotional and physical symptoms of caregiver burnout.

Take necessary precautions to relieve caregiver stress.

Share eldercare responsibilities with others.

PLAN ONE
Take an honest look at yourself.

Ask yourself the following questions to monitor your current caregiver stress level.
Do you . . .

Resent your elder? family members?
Find little satisfaction in assisting your aging relative?
Feel trapped and burdened?
Feel the rest of the family is not doing their share?
Have thoughts of guilt? shame? inadequacy? helplessness? hopelessness?
Have frequent feelings of anger or rage?
Maintain unrealistic attitudes? (I should . . .)
Think about being out of control? not being in control?
Have difficulty saying no to your aging relatives? to others?
Resist delegating eldercare responsibilities to others?

Are you . . .

Letting your job performance slip? late for work? missing work?
Using forms of physical abuse? verbal abuse?
Overeating? lacking an appetite? eating junk food?
Crying frequently?
Depleting your own financial resources?
Not seeking or accepting help?
Not asking questions or gathering information?
Not exercising? not having fun? not laughing?
Having fitful sleeping periods? nightmares?
Not sharing feelings?
Smoking? drinking? abusing drugs?
Developing physical symptoms like headaches, backaches, breathing problems,
    lingering colds?

PLAN TWO
Create relief.

There are people who will help care for your aging family members and people who will care for you. Ask for help, even if you don't perceive the need. The following is a list of people and organizations you may want to recruit:

> **Family, friends, neighbors, volunteers**—Let your needs be known. Call them now. Review this chapter's Share the Care section on page 31 for suggestions.

> **Employers**—Eldercare is fast replacing child care as the number one dependent-care workplace issue. Ask your employer about eldercare workshops and flex-time work options.

> **Support groups**—These groups meet regularly to discuss caregiving issues. Some programs provide education about particular illnesses, others may offer emotional support. Locate support groups through the local hospital discharge planner.

> **Specific illness associations**—Organizations dealing with specific illnesses such as cancer, diabetes, heart disease, arthritis, and Alzheimer's have programs for family members as well as patients.

PLAN THREE
Insist on family meetings and telephone conversations to bridge the care gap.

Regularly scheduled family meetings and telephone conversations between every member of the family is a practical way to address eldercare issues and delegate the responsibilities evenly.

If the elder is an aging parent, a common family problem arises when one child (most often a daughter), becomes the primary caregiver and resentment toward other siblings sets in. There are a variety of reasons why siblings do not do their share of eldercare:

- Parent wants only one child to care for him/her.
- Caregiver isn't asking for family members' help.
- Caregiver isn't assertive enough in demanding help from family members.

- Caregiver isn't willing to share the parent's attention with other family members.
- Sibling is in denial of what's happening and may choose to ignore the situation.
- Sibling lives far away and finds it difficult to help.
- Sibling feels overburdened with own responsibilities and is incapable of helping.
- Sibling contributes financially and feels that this is enough support.
- Male sibling may believe that caregiving is women's work.

The amount of assistance we receive from others is largely dependent on our willingness to ask for it. We are not the only one in the family who can provide care. We must share the responsibilities and insist on help from family members.

The most effective family meetings and telephone conversations employ clear and direct communication techniques. Limit agendas to a few important topics at one time. Give each family member equal time and allow the right to his/her opinion. Each must feel heard. Focus on the actions family members can take and resist the temptation to bring up ancient family history. Avoid accusatory statements and inappropriate expressions of anger. Instead of saying "You never help out . . ." you might say "I know you have a lot going on at work and it's hard for you, but do you think you can help me with . . ."

Most important, be specific about the kind of help you expect from family members. Don't beat around the bush. Say "I need your help and this is what I need . . ."

Low Cost/Free Resources

Contact the **State Department of Public Health** and the **State Mental Health Department** for information or assistance. Look in the **Government Agencies** section of the telephone book.

Refer to the telephone directory white pages under **Area Agency on Aging, American Red Cross, United Way, Catholic Charities, Family Service Agency, Visiting Nurses Association,** and **Jewish Family Services** for additional assistance.

For family caregivers providing home health care, many hospitals and adult education centers offer **home-nursing programs.**

The **Eldercare Locator** refers callers to an extensive network of organizations serving older people. Call toll-free (800) 677-1116. When you make your call, be prepared to provide the name, address, and zip code of your elder and a brief description of the problem or the kind of assistance you are seeking.

ORGANIZATIONS

American Association for Continuity of Care
638 Prospect Ave., Hartford, CT 06105, (203) 586-7525

American Society on Aging
833 Market St., San Francisco, CA 94103, (415) 974-9600, (800) 537-9728

Bureau of Elder & Adult Resource Directory
Website *http://www.state.me.us/beas/resource.htm*

Catholic Charities USA
1731 King St., Alexandria, VA 22314, (703) 549-1390
Website *http://ccsj.org/links.html*

Children of Aging Parents
1609 Woodburne Road, Suite 302A, Levittown, PA 19057, (215) 945-6900, (800) 227-7294

Christmas in April
1225 Eye St., NW, Washington, DC 20005, (202) 326-8268

Elder Support Network
PO Box 248, Kendall Park, NJ 08824, (800) 634-7346

Family Caregiver Alliance
425 Bush St., Suite 500, San Francisco, CA 94108, (415) 434-3388, (800) 445-8106

Family Resource Service
1400 Union Meeting Road, Suite 102, Blue Bell, PA 19422, (800) 847-5437

Foundation for Hospice and Home Care
519 C St., NE, Washington, DC 20002, (202) 547-6586

National Adult Day Care Services Association
c/o National Council on the Aging
409 Third St., SW, Suite 200, Washington, DC 20024, (202) 479-1200

National Association for Home Care
519 C St., NE, Washington, DC 20002, (202) 547-7424
Website *http://www.nahc.org*

National Association of Private Geriatric Case Managers
1604 N. Country Club Road, Tucson, AZ 85716, (520) 881-8008

National Center on Elder Abuse
810 First St., NE, Suite 500, Washington, DC 20002, (202) 682-2470

National Federation of Interfaith Volunteer Caregivers
PO Box 1939, Kingston, NY 12402, (914) 331-1358, (800) 350-7438

National Meals on Wheels Foundation
2675 44th St., SW, Suite 305, Grand Rapids, MI 49509, (616) 531-0090

Visiting Nurses Association of America
3801 E. Florida, Suite 900, Denver, CO 80210, (888) 866-8773

Volunteers of America, Inc.
3939 N. Causeway Blvd., Suite 400, Meairie, LA 70002, (800) 899-0089,
(504) 837-2652

Well Spouse Foundation
610 Lexington Ave., Suite 814, New York, NY 10022, (800) 838-0879,
(212) 644-1241

Action Checklist

HOW TO TELL WHEN YOUR ELDER NEEDS HELP	To Do By	Completed

Ask questions and observe elder's (Plan One) . . .

performing tasks	_____	❑
physical condition	_____	❑
environment	_____	❑
mental well-being	_____	❑

Discuss . . .

observations of elder	_____	❑
short-term solutions	_____	❑
long-term solutions	_____	❑

SHARE THE CARE

List eldercare tasks (Plan One) . . .

homemaker	_____	❑
personal care	_____	❑
home health care	_____	❑
quality of life	_____	❑

Set caregiver goals . . .

short-term	_____	❑
long-term	_____	❑

Make a caregiver list of who does what (Plan Two) . . .

short-term	_____	❑
long-term	_____	❑

Hire caregivers (Plan Four, Plan Five) . . .

create list of questions	_____	❑
create and sign job contract	_____	❑
check all references and licenses	_____	❑
have proper insurance	_____	❑
look into Social Security taxes	_____	❑

Have a plan to (Plan Six, Plan Seven) . . .

oversee quality of care   _____   ❑

get updates on elder's condition   _____   ❑

praise caregivers   _____   ❑

report elder abuse   _____   ❑

Review community programs (Plan Eight) . . .

home-delivered meals   _____   ❑

emergency response devices   _____   ❑

carrier alert   _____   ❑

social day care   _____   ❑

adult day health care   _____   ❑

respite care   _____   ❑

Consider volunteers (Plan Nine) . . .   _____   ❑

Obtain a copy of elder's . . .

telephone directory   _____   ❑

personal address book   _____   ❑

community senior directory   _____   ❑

Record emergency telephone numbers.   _____   ❑

Know phone numbers of . . .

hospital social services   _____   ❑

family service agency   _____   ❑

area agency on aging   _____   ❑

Visiting Nurses Association   _____   ❑

family members   _____   ❑

elder's neighbors and friends   _____   ❑

co-workers   _____   ❑

caregivers   _____   ❑

geriatric case manager   _____   ❑

social worker   _____   ❑

Make sure elder has access to a telephone.   _____   ❑

Duplicate and file phone numbers. Keep copies . . .

at home   _____   ❑

at work   _____   ❑

    in car   _____ ❑

    in wallet/purse   _____ ❑

Duplicate and distribute phone numbers to designated persons.   _____ ❑

TAKE CARE OF YOU

Create self-care goals . . .

    short-term   _____ ❑

    long-term   _____ ❑

Monitor caregiver stress (Plan One).   _____ ❑

Plan for caregiver relief (Plan Two) . . .

    schedule days off   _____ ❑

    support groups   _____ ❑

    vacations   _____ ❑

    maintain personal interests   _____ ❑

    community respite programs   _____ ❑

Organize regular family meetings and telephone conversations (Plan Three).   _____ ❑

Chapter 3

EMERGENCY PREPAREDNESS

Quick and Easy Access

Planning ahead does family caregivers little good if they don't have twenty-four-hour accessibility to their aging relatives and their property. Imagine not being able to reach your family member because you don't have the key to his/her home. Or you meant to give an extra set of keys to your elder's neighbor but you never got around to it. Do you know who will call an ambulance if you are unreachable when an emergency arises?

The absence of legal documents is another extremely stressful situation for family members. For instance, if your elder is temporarily incapacitated and you do not have power of attorney for his/her checking account, you may have to spend your own money in the interim to pay your relative's bills.

Inaccessibility complicates the caregiving process. This section of the planner will show you how this situation can *easily* be avoided. The process of duplicating keys, creating check-in systems, implementing legal documents, arranging for financial access, and obtaining emergency telephone numbers prepares you to the best of your abilities for any eldercare crisis that might arise.

QUICK AND EASY ACCESS

• In an emergency, minutes count . . . and getting help
could make the difference between life and death.

**If your aging relative is alone and an emergency occurs, you have
the satisfaction of knowing someone is always close at hand.**

Objectives

After completing Quick and Easy Access you will be able to:

Assist aging family members twenty-four hours a day, seven
days a week.

Create access to your elder and your elder's property in an emergency.

PLAN ONE

Keep important telephone numbers handy.

Record the names and telephone numbers of your relative's emergency contacts. Use the form provided in this planner on page 3. If time is limited, photocopy his/her personal address book. Make copies of this list of contacts and distribute to your elder, other family members, friends, co-workers, and neighbors.

Keep a copy of this list at home and at work. Post the list near the telephone or on the refrigerator at your home and your elder's home. Keep a copy in your wallet or purse. Update names and phone numbers as needed.

Obtain a copy of your relative's community telephone directories—white pages and yellow pages. If your relative lives outside of your 911 emergency district, you must call the police or fire department directly. Look these numbers up ahead of time and write them down.

PLAN TWO

Gain twenty-four-hour access to your elder and elder's property.

Duplicate keys, plastic access cards, electronic openers, and combinations. Label keys and selectively distribute to family, friends, and neighbors. Maintain twenty-four-hour access to keys and to those having access. Distribute keys in person if possible. If your family member has voice mail on the telephone and E-mail on the computer, learn the access code in order to retrieve messages.

To draw money from your relative's checking and savings accounts, most banks require power of attorney prearranged on *their* forms. Another strategy is to set up a second signature on designated accounts. To make either one of these financial arrangements, accompany your elder to the bank and fill out the appropriate forms. NOTE: If a safe deposit key is given to someone whose signature is not on file, that person will not have access to the box.

To locate key duplicating services, see the yellow pages under Locks and Locksmiths. Duplicate keys for . . .

Residence	Bicycle	Mailbox	Storage
Garage	Other vehicles	Office	Personal business safe
Gate	R.V./Boat	Desk	Luggage/Trunk
Auto	Trailer	Alarm	Locks

PLAN THREE
Make alternate plans if aging family members choose to keep total control of their property and money.

Ask your elder to disclose the names and telephone numbers of those who have access to property and legal documents. Write this information down in the Documents Locator section starting on page 229 so you will know who to call in an emergency.

PLAN FOUR
Create check-in systems.

Ideally, your elder will be able to use the telephone to call for help when an emergency occurs. However, this is often not the case. Make contact with aging family members on a regular basis by phone, in person, or with the use of beepers. Create a network of people who agree to stay in touch with your elder. See Chapter Eight, Safe and Secure, page 156 for a variety of check-in options.

PLAN FIVE
Consider the protection of a medical alert system.

Identification of hidden medical conditions saves lives in an emergency. Simple options like printed, wallet-size cards and identification bracelets and necklaces are adequate. Call the area agency on aging and the hospital discharge planner for recommendations. Hidden medical conditions include . . .

Diabetes	Hypertension	Drug usage	Hemodialysis
Asthma	Pacemaker	Cateracts	Organ donor
Emphysema	Angina	Hyperthermia	Osteoporosis
Epilepsy	Alzheimer's	Hypoglycemia	Hepatitis
Glaucoma	Coronary bypass	Hemophilia	Osteoarthritis
Implants	Allergies	Contact lenses	Heart disease

PLAN SIX
Keep copies of vital information at home, at work, in your wallet or purse.

Compile the following information regarding your aging family member and update as needed:

Emergency telephone numbers	Durable power of attorney for health care
Blood type	Durable power of attorney
Medical conditions	Driver's license
Medications	Allergies
Social Security number	Proof of insurance

Managing Medications

Over-the-counter drugs and prescription drugs are both serious medicines. Aging people also may be under the care of several different doctors at the same time, each doctor possibly prescribing different medications. Every year close to 125,000 people die from taking the wrong medicine, the wrong dosage, or taking the drugs improperly.

If your relative is taking *any* medication, this is one caregiving issue that cannot be ignored. This section of the planner offers specific guidelines on becoming familiar with your elder's drug usage and action plans that prevent deadly medication mishaps.

Self-medication with over-the-counter drugs also has emerged as an important component to health maintenance for older adults. This allows them to take greater control over their own health care. Encourage aging family members to be educated consumers. Reading labels, following directions, asking questions, and taking proper amounts of the drug are essential elements of managing medications responsibly.

MANAGING MEDICATIONS

- A Food and Drug Administration (FDA) report found that people seventy years and older fill an average of thirteen prescriptions per year. Some of these people may fill as many as fourteen to eighteen different prescriptions in a one-year period.
- Studies indicate that patients in nursing homes may be taking as many as thirty medications.

If your aging family members are taking medications, your involvement in fact-finding and safety precautions could very well prevent serious mishaps, including death.

Objectives

*After completing **Managing Medications** you will be able to:*

Know what purpose each prescription serves.

Establish a doctor/elder/pharmacist relationship.

Uncover the possibility of mismanagement of drugs.

Assist your elder in managing his/her medications responsibly.

PLAN ONE
Investigate which drugs your elder is taking and why.

Get involved. It is imperative that your relative's health-care providers are aware that others are monitoring medical procedures and prescriptions. Intervention saves lives. If your family member cannot or does not want to answer questions regarding medications to your satisfaction, it is time to step in.

Ask your elder . . .

What medicine are you taking?
What is the medicine supposed to do?

Review with your elder and your elder's doctor alternative methods of treating your relative's condition without the use of drugs—weight loss, special diet, exercise, massage therapy, bed rest, and ice packs, for example.

If you suspect that your elder's doctor's prescription policy automatically includes drugs as a way to cope with life's expected conditions, such as bereavement, you may want to suggest switching doctors.

PLAN TWO
Is your elder overmedicated? Find out.

Aging family members who are attended to by several doctors may neglect telling each one about the drugs being prescribed by the other. To lower dangerous levels of drug usage and to prevent deadly drug combinations, inform each prescriber of all routinely used medications, including over-the-counter drugs and vitamins.

"Brown-bag it." Gather your elder's medications, prescription drugs, and over-the-counter medications including eye drops, cough syrup, pain relievers, cold pills, and vitamins and put them in a paper bag. Take them to your elder's next doctor's appointment or to the pharmacist for a review.

Have your elder's prescriptions filled at only one pharmacy. The pharmacist will keep track of drug usage by computer and can easily track the possibility of overmedication and dangerous drug combinations.

Create a drug-usage chart to bring to every appointment. Photocopy charts ahead of time. Record current drug and over-the-counter drug usage information. Complete new prescription information in the doctor's office. NOTE: If you think this is too much trouble, be assured that intervention saves lives. Any physician or assistant who avoids answering questions or gives family members little time to ask questions should be viewed with suspicion.

DRUG USAGE CHART

Drug Name	Drug Purpose	Drug Color & Shape	Amount to Take	When to Take	How to Take	How Long to Take	Possible Side Effects

PLAN THREE
Know the reasons why elderly patients may not follow prescription directions.

Elders sometimes discontinue, resume, or change medications without the physician's consent, which can be quite harmful. The reasons include . . .

• The drugs make them feel worse than the symptoms of the illness.
• There is no clear evidence that the drug is working.

• Medications are too expensive.
• They would rather spend their money on something else.
• They feel better.
• Taking drugs gives them a feeling of loss of independence.
• Drugs are a constant reminder of "being sick."
• Short-term memory makes it hard to track drug usage.

PLAN FOUR
Get the most from the pharmacist.

A certified pharmacist, registered with the state pharmaceutical board, is highly trained to answer questions about drugs.

Ask the pharmacist . . .

• Any questions regarding drugs.
• If generic drugs are available.
• For written information about the medicine.
• To keep a file on the elder's drug usage and medical history.
• For easy-open containers as long as there are no children present.
• About senior citizen discounts.
• For large-print labels.
• About twenty-four-hour telephone and emergency services.
• About prescription home-delivery services.
• About year-end tax and insurance statements.

PLAN FIVE
Explore the possibility that your relative may be taking medicines improperly.

Make sure that your elder knows the answers to these important questions . . .

What medicine am I taking?
What will the medicine do for me?
How should I take it?
When should I take it?

How will I know the medicine is working?

How long will it take the medicine to work?

How long must I take this drug?

What are the expected side effects?

Can I relieve these side effects?

Is it safe to drink alcohol?

What foods should be avoided?

Will the use of over-the-counter drugs be harmful?

Will taking multiple medications be a dangerous combination?

Is it okay to crush pills or even dissolve them in water?

Will smoking, coffee, or caffeinated beverages cause reactions?

What activities (driving, operating machinery) should be avoided?

Is exposure to sunlight harmful?

What is the shelf life of the drug?

How should the drug be stored?

Can I switch to generic drugs?

Are there sexual side effects when taking this drug?

Can the medicine cause an allergic reaction?

What should I do if I forget to take the medicine?

What will happen if I do not take the medicine?

PLAN SIX
Implement on-going drug safety precautions.

Discuss and implement the following options:

- If forgetfulness is a problem for your elder, create a chart. List the days of the week, the name of each medication, the times to take each drug, then cross out the drug each time it is taken.
- If your relative plans on using a plastic pill box (found at most drugstores), keep the original prescription container handy. Keep a sample of each drug in its original container. When traveling, pack the original drug container as well.
- Make sure the prescription labels are clear and in large print. Keep a magnifying glass near prescription containers. If your elder wears glasses, remind him/her to wear them when reading labels.

- Use pharmacist-provided colored containers for different drugs.
- When filling prescriptions, check the name of the drug on the label before leaving the pharmacy.
- Don't mix alcohol and drugs.
- Consult the doctor before taking over-the-counter drugs.
- Ask party hosts if the food or beverages they are serving contain alcohol.
- Store drugs as directed. Refrigerate the drug only if told to do so.
- Know the expected side effects of the drugs.
- Never share drugs. Never.
- Keep pills a distance from bed. This reduces the possibility of taking the wrong dose or wrong combination when sleepy. Do not take drugs in the dark.
- Read labels in properly lighted rooms.
- Discard medicines that have expired or have no labels.
- Ask the doctor or pharmacist if the drug is habit-forming.
- Ask the doctor to order a home visit from a nurse to teach the elder how to manage medications.
- Discuss the fact that making rapid movements like standing up too quickly can cause unnecessary falls.
- Ask your family member to keep a list of drugs in use, prescription and over-the-counter, in his/her wallet or purse at all times.
- Keep a list of drugs in use on the refrigerator or by the telephone.
- Do business with just one reliable pharmacy.
- Keep each doctor informed of all prescriptions.
- Share written medication information with every family member.
- Check with the doctor before asking the pharmacist to substitute generic drugs for the prescription.
- Make use of identification bracelets for allergies and chronic conditions.
- Before purchasing over-the-counter drugs, examine the packages for signs of tampering. If the seal is broken or it looks like the box has been opened, get another package and return the damaged one to the store manager.

If Your Elder Is Hospitalized

Every hospital and medical center has a culture all its own. Family caregivers who have little experience in dealing with health-care professionals in these specialized environments too often don't know what to expect, what to do, or what questions to ask. From the moment you arrive at the hospital, feelings of confusion and fear are normal, especially if your relative is taken there unexpectedly.

No matter the circumstance, this section of the planner provides immediate action plans that help you gain control over an emergency situation. Hospitalization is a traumatic experience for the entire family. Surviving this stressful situation requires asking specific questions and making informed decisions based on facts, not emotions. Veteran caregivers will tell you that a crash course on planning, organizing, and communication skills is in order. The good news is, you are holding the manual in your hands.

IF YOUR ELDER IS HOSPITALIZED

- Asking specific questions and making decisions based on facts, not overwhelming emotions, is the key to managing your elder's hospitalization.
- The law gives patients the right to refuse care or treatment at any time.
- The reality of health care today means that people are whisked in and out of the hospital in record time. A typical stay is under one week.

It is possible to take a proactive stance if your family member is admitted to the hospital and to be prepared for hasty hospital discharges.

Objectives

After completing If Your Elder Is Hospitalized you will be able to:

Ask revealing questions during times of confusion.

Gather important health-care information and legal documents.

Make your elder's hospital stay as comfortable as possible.

Research home and institutional health-care options.

Plan ahead for your relative's needs after his/her hospitalization.

PLAN ONE
Be proactive.

Create an eldercare file on your relative. Include a legal-size pad of paper in this file to write down questions, answers, phone numbers, things to do. Put dates on your notes. Save all documentation, reports, lab tests, bills, notes, and anything related to your family member's hospitalization. Save receipts on money you spend for possible reimbursement from your elder, the insurance company, other family members, settlements, or taxes.

Also keep copies of your elder's proof of health insurance and the **living will, durable power of attorney,** and **durable power of attorney for health care** in this file. See Chapter Five, Legal Matters, page 103, for more information on these documents.

Attach copies of the living will and the durable power of attorney for health care to your **elder's medical chart.**

If your family member is too ill to speak and has not left instructions in a living will regarding medical treatment, the law requires the hospital staff to administer every treatment they deem appropriate to keep the patient alive.

Keep your elder's file folder with you everywhere you go as long as he/she is hospitalized. You may need it at a moment's notice.

PLAN TWO
Take it one step at a time.

With so many questions and so many things to do, you may be overwhelmed to the point of doing nothing or doing too much with little direction. Follow the action plans in this chapter in the order shown. Go at your own pace.

To begin, make a heading called Elder Contacts on the first page of your pad of paper or write information down in the space provided here. List the names, addresses, and phone numbers (day and evening) of the individuals suggested in the lists below. Record this information as soon as you make contact with these people.

If an accident occurred . . .

    Police on duty   Insurance agents
    Accident victims   Lawyer

At the hospital . . .

Hospital and hospital address
Hospital floor, room, and bed number
Nurses
Head nurse
Doctor(s)

Specialists
Social worker
Discharge planner
Patient representative
Billing director

Caregiver support . . .

Family
Friends
Neighbors
Volunteers
Area agency on aging

Family service agency
Public health department
Home health-care agencies
Geriatric case manager
Visiting Nurses Association

Posthospital recovery . . .

Board and care facility
Skilled nursing facility
Home hospital equipment

Adult day care
24-hour Pharmacy

Home management . . .

Housekeeper
House sitter
Pet sitter

Handyman
Home chore services

Business . . .

Co-workers
Insurance agents
Lawyers

Accountant
Banker
Social Security office

Personal . . .

Beauty care
Clubs/Associations

Church
Volunteer activity

PLAN THREE

Know what questions to ask doctors and nurses.

If your family member is unable to communicate and is in serious condition, and a living will or durable power of attorney for health care has been prepared in advance, now is the time to review the contents. If you are the designated agent who is responsible for deciding your relative's medical treatment, seek the advice of the family doctor, the hospital social worker, and a member of the clergy. With their help you can gather the facts about your elder's condition. If health care directives have not been secured in advance, ask to be informed of your rights as a decision-making family member.

As you encounter medical personnel, jot down names, phone numbers, questions and answers on your pad of paper. Date your notes.

Ask medical providers . . .

Is my family member in any immediate danger?
What is the medical problem?
What are the short-term effects of this illness?
What are the long-term effects of this illness?
Will my family member stay in the hospital now? How long?
What medications have been prescribed?

If surgery is recommended, ask . . .

What are the possible complications?
What are the short-term expectations?
What are the long-term expectations?
What happens if my elder does not have the surgery?
How often do you perform this procedure?
What is the success rate?
What is the rate of complications from this surgery?
Is surgery needed now or can it wait?
What are the other choices of treatment?
What are the short-term consequences if surgery is not performed?
What are the long-term consequences if surgery is not performed?
(If surgery is recommended remind yourself of the second-opinion option.)

If your elder is to be released from the hospital, ask . . .

Will my elder need home health care assistance? What kind?
Where will this help come from?
Is this care covered by insurance?
What is the expected recovery time?

If your elder is staying overnight in the hospital, ask elder . . .

Is there anyone specifically you would like me to contact?
Is there anything you would like me to bring you?

Plan Four
Be prepared for the enormous task of making telephone calls.

There will be many phone calls to make and many questions to answer. You will tell your elder's story over and over again. Friends and family members will want to know every detail. Be prepared to hear some of their own medical experiences—be patient; once they finish with their stories, you can get down to business. There also may be rumors and gossip you have to extinguish.

Don't promise to keep everyone informed of your elder's progress (except a select few). You will have enough to do. Instead, ask that they call you back.

Well-meaning family and friends will ask you about telephoning and visiting your relative in the hospital. Give them clear instructions if you or your elder do not want to be disturbed; but don't be surprised if they call and visit anyway.

The task of making telephone calls is extremely overwhelming. It is very important that you delegate and share this responsibility with other reliable people. Do not underestimate the pressures of this task.

Locate your elder's personal address book and appointment book. Make copies of both for the purpose of making calls. Calls to make:

Accident-related calls . . .

Police	Lawyer
Insurance agents	Witnesses

Cancel your elder's activities . . .

Employment	Volunteer
Appointments	Social commitments

Meetings	Travel
Ongoing commitments	Engagements
Carpools	Classes

Suspend . . .

| Newspaper delivery | Mail pickup, and make other arrangements |

Call . . .

Family	Insurance Agent
Friends	Church group
Neighbors	Clergy
Business relations	Housekeeping services
Landlord	House sitter
Accountant/Banker	Pet sitter
Lawyer	Homes-chores person

PLAN FIVE

Make a list of business to take care of while your elder is in the hospital.

Before you leave the hospital, be sure to take your elder's valuables (watch, jewelry, wallet, purse) home with you. Store them in a safe place. Review the following suggestions as a way to take care of family business in the meantime.

At elder's home . . .

• Retrieve messages from the telephone answering machine, voice mail, or E-mail.
• Follow up on important calls.
• Make a list of phone calls to make (See Plan Four).
• Locate your elder's personal address and appointment book. Keep this book with you, if possible, or make copies.
• Find proof of your elder's health insurance. Record the policy name and number. Keep a copy of the insurance card in your folder file.
• Go through the mail. Pay urgent bills.
• Keep track of money spent on eldercare for possible reimbursement.
• Notify creditors and let them know your elder is in the hospital.

- Make duplicate keys to the home, property, auto, and mailbox.
- Make bank deposits on elder's behalf.
- Pack items to bring back with you to the hospital (See Plan Six).
- Go through the refrigerator and throw out spoiled foods. Take home the rest.
- Check and maintain the security of home and auto.
- Store valuables, jewelry, wallet, purse, credit cards, and driver's license in a safe place.
- Make living arrangements for his/her spouse if necessary.
- If it's near tax time, locate the tax file or contact the accountant for an extension.
- Pack up medications and show them to the doctor at the hospital.
- Have mail picked up regularly or put on hold at the post office.
- Suspend newspapers that are home delivered.
- Have lawn mowed, snow shoveled.

At your home . . .

- Make phone calls (See Plan Four).
- Get cash and change for the telephone or carry your telephone calling card.
- Pack for overnight visits.
- Make home, work, and personal arrangements.

PLAN SIX
Make your elder's hospital stay as comfortable as possible.

Ask what items you can bring back with you to the hospital. Suggest:

Favorite pajamas	Robe
Slippers	Toothbrush
Shaver/Shaving lotion	Hairbrush/Comb
Self-standing mirror	Hand/Body/Face lotion
Perfume	Lipstick
Makeup	Nail care kit
Deodorant	Personal address book
Appointment book	Handicraft project
Laptop games/Computer	Books/Magazines

Transistor/Walkman radio	Hearing aid
Glasses/Glasses cleaner	Crossword puzzles
Paper/Pen/Stationery	Stuffed animal
Chewing gum/Mints	Snacks/Food *(if diet allows)*
Street clothes/Shoes/Socks	Undergarments

PLAN SEVEN
Plan ahead as elder recuperates in the hospital.

You will need to make decisions regarding home or institutionalized health care *before* your elder is released from the hospital. Seek assistance from the hospital discharge planner about home and health-care options early on. Hospitals release patients sooner than you think and it is best to be prepared as soon as possible.

Laws state that patients are free to leave the hospital upon release from their doctor. The hospital is not allowed to detain patients who have outstanding medical expenses and fees not covered by their health insurance carrier.

Ask the doctor . . .

Will home nursing care be needed? Full-time? Part-time?
What other kind of care will be needed? Short-term? Long-term?
What lifestyle changes are expected?
What symptoms could indicate health complications?

Ask the hospital discharge planner . . .

Who can I call to get home health-care assistance?
What are the options for living arrangements during recuperation?
What hospital and home-care costs are covered by insurance?

Review elder's living-arrangement options . . .

• Elder's home
• Family's home
• Friend's home
• Board and care facility
• Intermediate care facility
• Skilled nursing facility

Review home-care options (see Chapter Two, Caregivers, page 31) . . .

• Visiting nurse
• Nurses aide
• Family
• Friends
• Homemaker services
• Social day care
• Adult day health care
• Volunteer

Review elder's needs (see Chapter Two, Caregivers, page 26) . . .

• Homemaker services
• Personal care
• Home health care
• Quality of life

PLAN EIGHT
Use the services of the hospital patient representative.

Patient representatives assist family members with their elders' health-care problems, concerns, and unmet needs that may have occurred during the hospital stay. Representatives serve as a liaison between patients and the hospital administration.

• The patient representative . . .
• Evaluates the level of patient satisfaction.
• Channels information about care problems to appropriate departments.
• Directs inquiries and complaints to appropriate hospital staff.
• Refers patients to services and resources.
• Investigates patient care complaints.
• Assesses responses to incidents.

Low Cost/Free Resources

To learn **CPR** (cardiopulmonary resuscitation) find classes by calling the YMCA, the local fire station, the American Heart Association, or the American Red Cross. Check the yellow pages under **First Aid Instruction.**

Telecommunication devices for the deaf (TDD) and **Braille TDDs** are available for telephone customers with hearing and sight disabilities. Contact the Special Needs Center of the telephone company.

Carrier alert, also known as postal alert, is a volunteer program in which letter carriers monitor the possible need of emergency services when they examine mail that has not been removed from mailboxes. For more information, contact the area agency on aging or the post office. Also see Chapter Eight, Safe and Secure, page 149.

ORGANIZATIONS

American Heart Association National Center and Stroke Connection
7272 Greenville Ave., Dallas, TX 75231, (800) 242-8721, (800) 553-6321 (for stroke-related questions), (214) 373-6300

American Red Cross
430 17th St., NW, Washington, DC 20006, (202) 737-8300
Website *http://www.crossnet.org/triangle/otherarc.htm*

American Trauma Society
8903 Presidential Parkway, Suite 512, Upper Marlboro, MD 20772, (800) 556-7890, (301) 420-4189

Council on Family Health
225 Park Ave. South, Suite 1700, New York, NY 10003, (212) 598-3617

National Clearinghouse for Alcohol and Drug Information
(800) 729-6686

Action Checklist

QUICK AND EASY ACCESS	To Do By	Completed
Set elder access goals . . .		
short-term	_____	❏
long-term	_____	❏
Know the twenty-four-hour emergency phone numbers (Plan One) . . .		
doctor(s)	_____	❏
dentist	_____	❏
neighbors	_____	❏
friends	_____	❏
police	_____	❏
fire	_____	❏
hospital	_____	❏
hospice	_____	❏
nurse	_____	❏
home aide	_____	❏
pharmacist	_____	❏
electrician	_____	❏
plumber	_____	❏
water company	_____	❏
gas company	_____	❏
electric company	_____	❏
telephone company	_____	❏
alarm company	_____	❏
locksmith	_____	❏
clergy	_____	❏
Keep copies of emergency phone numbers . . .		
at home	_____	❏
at work	_____	❏
in car	_____	❏
in wallet/purse	_____	❏

QUICK AND EASY ACCESS	To Do By	Completed
Give copies of emergency phone numbers to key people.	_____	❑
Duplicate keys (Plan Two).	_____	❑
Identify and store keys and openers.	_____	❑
Distribute keys to key people.	_____	❑
Have a plan to access finances in an emergency (Plan Two).	_____	❑
Have a backup plan if access to finances is denied (Plan Three).	_____	❑
Consider a medical alert system (Plan Five).	_____	❑
Create a check-in system (Plan Four).	_____	❑
Elder has access to a telephone.	_____	❑

MANAGING MEDICATIONS

Discuss medications with . . .

	To Do By	Completed
elder	_____	❑
doctor	_____	❑
pharmacist (Plan Three)	_____	❑
family members	_____	❑

Discuss drug . . .

	To Do By	Completed
usage (Plans One, Three)	_____	❑
purpose (Plans One, Three)	_____	❑
alternatives (Plan One)	_____	❑
safety (Plans Five, Six)	_____	❑

	To Do By	Completed
Create drug chart (Plan Two).	_____	❑
Schedule a CPR class.	_____	❑

IF YOUR ELDER IS HOSPITALIZED

Start a file folder (Plan One). _____ ❑

Create a system for recording and filing . . .
    phone numbers (Plan Two) _____ ❑
    community resources _____ ❑
    helpers _____ ❑
    eldercare receipts _____ ❑
    notes/documentation _____ ❑
    bills _____ ❑
    questions/answers _____ ❑

Create list of questions for medical providers
(Plans Three, Seven). _____ ❑

Review care options (Plan Seven). _____ ❑

Make phone calls (Plan Four). _____ ❑

Review things to do (Plan Five). _____ ❑

Ask what to bring to hospital (Plan Six). _____ ❑

Chapter 4

MONEY MATTERS

The Cost of Caring

The financial considerations of assisting aging relatives run deep—we spend our money to cover eldercare expenses such as home care, groceries, and travel. Some family caregivers take time off work to help out, which impacts their spending capabilities even more. At the same time, the decreasing eligibility and benefits of government programs such as Medicare and Medicaid are altering the economic conditions of our elderly for the worse. Medicare provides very limited payments for long-term care and Medicaid won't pay for nursing home care until the elder's funds are nearly depleted. Overall, if we do not plan for the business side of caregiving, the family's financial resources may suffer serious consequences.

Consider the hidden costs of eldercare. Long-distance telephone bills add up quickly. Then there are times when we arrive at our relative's home and notice that a leaky faucet needs fixing, or that the food supply is low, or a prescription needs to be filled. The necessity to run to the hardware store, grocery store, and the pharmacy is an all-too-common economic predicament. As a result of continuously dipping into our own pockets we soon run out of money.

We want to be helpful, but we sabotage these intentions when we do not maintain our own financial stability or are unaware of the costs that lie ahead. If you are or will be assisting an aging family member and spending your own money in the process, this section of the planner prepares you for the cost of caring and offers plans to avoid a personal financial disaster.

THE COST OF CARING

- Long-distance assistance adds up. Family caregivers can expect to spend money on travel, telephone bills, lodging, and much more.
- Aging parents may wish their children to believe that the family finances are in better shape than they actually are.
- The American Association for Continuity of Care reports that as many as 40 percent of older Americans have incomes of less than $6,000 per year, having less—or choosing to spend less—than $25 to $30 per week for food.

The sooner family caregivers understand the impact of eldercare on their own hard-earned money, the better their chances for long-term financial stability.

Objectives

After completing The Cost of Caring you will be able to:

Be aware of the cost of eldercare.

Calculate and budget for short- and long-term expenses.

Create opportunities for everyone to pitch in.

PLAN ONE
Pay attention to the business side of caregiving.

We may find ourselves in the position of supplementing the cost of a wide variety of products and services needed by our aging family members. Some items are very expensive like home health care and housing. Don't underestimate, however, the hidden costs of caring. It's the "little things" that add up. The following lists serve as a guide for calculating eldercare expenditures:

Elder's home expenses . . .

- Interior and exterior maintenance *(housekeeping, yard work)*
- Home and appliance repairs
- Remodeling *(first-floor bathroom and bedroom, clothes closets)*
- Modifications *(door widths, ramps, lighting sources, shelf and counter heights)*
- Fixtures *(handrails, lifting platforms, door levers, locks, window cranks)*

Household items to purchase . . .

- Cordless telephones
- Telephone answering machine *(voice mail)*
- Automatic on/off appliances
- Adjustable furniture and bed
- Remote-control devices
- Bathroom fixtures *(shower stool, raised toilet seat, grab bar)*
- Nonbreakable glasses and dishware

Basic living expenses . . .

- Groceries
- Housing *(rent, monthly payments)*
- Utilities *(heat, air-conditioning, electricity, water, telephone)*
- Clothes and footwear
- Transportation
- Assisted-living services *(bathing, dressing, shopping, cooking, errands)*
- Beauty care *(hairdresser, manicure, pedicure)*
- Travel
- Entertainment *(cable television services)*

Home health-care expenses ...

• Nursing services
• Medications *(prescriptions, over-the-counter drugs, vitamins)*
• Special diets
• Emergency paging systems *(call buttons)*
• Home hospital equipment
• Walkers, canes, wheelchairs
• Hearing aid, glasses prescriptions

Caring from a distance costs family members plenty. Whether you are traveling from the next town or across the ocean, if assisting your relative means physically being there, these are the expenses to consider for making the trip.

Travel expenses ...

• Airfare *(ask each airline about its policy for emergency family travel)*
• Ground transportation *(bus, train, taxi, limo)*
• Car rental
• Car gas
• Tolls
• En route *(food, lodging)*

Home expenses ...

• Child care
• House sitter
• Pet sitter

Destination expenses ...

• Food
• Lodging
• Parking
• Long-distance telephone calls

PLAN TWO
Can you afford eldercare? Find out.

To budget for short- and long-term eldercare expenses, consider your personal economic situation, the realistic ability to make financial contributions, and your attitude about spending your own money on such expenditures. Ask yourself the following questions:

> *What is my short-term financial picture? Long-term?*
> *How much can I afford?*
> *How much of my own money and resources am I willing to spend?*

To make eldercare financing more efficient, keep a written record of important information. In addition to assets and liabilities, your financial plan should also note the location of valuable papers and property. See Chapter Thirteen, Documents Locator, page 229. If you are employed outside the home, you must also figure into the equation any lost income from missing work due to on-site eldercare responsibilities. Consider the following for your eldercare budget:

Your current and future assets . . .

- Income *(salary, pensions, interest income, IRAs, tax shelters, Social Security)*
- Investment income *(property, stocks, bonds, mutual funds)*
- Assets *(property, collectibles, valuables)*
- Annuities *(surrender value)*
- Bank accounts *(checking, savings, credit unions, money markets, certificates of deposit, cash on hand)*
- Income tax returns
- Loans receivable *(IOUs to you)*
- Business equity

Your current and future liabilities . . .

- Insurance policies *(life, health, disability, home, auto)*
- Credit cards
- Mortgages, debts, loans *(what is owed, when payments are due)*
- Child support/Alimony
- Child care
- Education
- Miscellaneous obligations

PLAN THREE
Who pays for what?

The question of how much of our own money we are willing to spend is a complicated and difficult one to answer. Some families feel as if they are required to "spend into poverty" to qualify for government programs like Medicaid.

When nursing home care is required, the cost of this level of care is giving family members sticker shock. Most American families cannot afford decent long-term care insurance, much less nursing home costs.

Taking on eldercare expenses could be an impossible burden for many. Family members who are already doing their share to pay for the bills of their older relatives ask: *How will we finance the affairs of our own family?* and *How are we going to retire if the money we have saved is sufficient for us, but may not be sufficient if we have to help with the bills of our elderly relatives?*

One solution is the theory of estate recovery, a program that basically goes after the house of beneficiaries after they die. Rather than asking family members to pay long-term care costs, some eldercare advocates are asking that government policies beef up estate-recovery laws.

Seek the professional advice of an estate-planning attorney, a certified financial planner, and a trusted insurance agent who will assist the family with short- and long-term eldercare financial goals.

PLAN FOUR
Ask for help with time and money.

After you have explored the costs associated with assisting your aging family member and examined your present and future financial situation, the next step is to create opportunities for everyone to pitch in.

To get an idea of your elder's financial stability to handle his/her expenses, review the next section in this chapter, Ready Cash, starting on page 85.

Now is the time to develop a family plan for current and future eldercare expenses:

• Create eldercare savings and checking accounts. Set money aside in these accounts as much as your budget allows. Ask other family members to do the same.

- Initiate conversations with your family members regarding reimbursement policies from your relative's estate, insurance company, tax deductions, and any legal settlements. Keep all receipts.
- Reevaluate you elder's financial needs every six months.

Ask the entire family to give in terms of time and resources:

- Interior and exterior home repairs
- Home maintenance
- Housekeeping
- Laundry
- Heavy lifting
- Shopping and errands
- Transportation
- Cooking
- Personal care
- Paying bills
- Managing medications
- Social activities
- Exercise
- Religious interests

Ready Cash

Until very recently, bringing up the subject of money with your elders was considered off-limits by family members. Your relatives may have assumed that the state of their finances was private information and we assumed that they were living within their means and that there might even be money and property to inherit after they died.

Today, people are living to be very old and the costs associated with a longer life can easily wipe out the entire family's financial resources. The money conversation taboo needs to be lifted. Family members have the right to initiate financial discussions with their aging relatives since they are typically the ones who must step in and pick up the tab when the resources run dry.

It is never too early or too late to initiate money conversations. The most important thing to do is to simply get started. This section of the planner is designed to help you review, budget, and access financial resources. Express love and concern for your elders' safety and enjoyment in later years when you ask that they share financial information for the sake of your honoring their future wishes.

READY CASH

- The average life span for men and women has increased. Elders have to support themselves for about a third longer than they thought they would.
- Most chronic long-term illnesses are not covered by Medicare. When an aging person can no longer afford these bills, the children are typically the ones who pick up the tab.
- The family's first defense against disability should be a large emergency fund.

If your aging relative is financially close to the edge, you can ease the strain without diminishing respect or depriving your own family of needed financial resources.

Objectives

*After completing **Ready Cash** you will be able to:*

Review your elder's present financial status.

Determine the existence of a deficit.

Assist in financial planning.

Protect the entire family's finances for the long run.

PLAN ONE
Help your elder plan for financial fitness.

Review your elder's current financial state. Use the budget worksheet below to track income and expenses.

AVERAGE MONTHLY INCOME

Salary/wages/commissions _____
Interest & Dividends _____
Social Security _____
IRA/Keogh _____
Pension/Profit Sharing _____
Rental Income _____
Other _____

TOTAL INCOME $ _____

AVERAGE MONTHLY EXPENSES

Housing—rent or mortgage _____
    Taxes _____
    Insurance _____
    Maintenance/Repairs _____
    Utilities _____
Food/Tobacco/Alcohol _____
Automobile Payments _____
    Maintenance/Repairs _____
    License/Fees _____
    Medical Insurance _____
Clothing _____
Health Care _____
    Medical Insurance _____
Personal Care _____
Other Insurance _____
Entertainment _____
Travel _____
Gifts/Contributions _____
Other _____

TOTAL EXPENSES $ _____

TOTAL INCOME $ _____
SUBTRACT TOTAL EXPENSES $ _____
MONTHLY BALANCE $ _____

PLAN TWO
Reduce your elder's debts and living expenses.

Make these suggestions to help your family member gain control of spending:

- Keep a daily written account of any money spent.
- Purchase low-maintenance products.
- Buy only what's on sale.
- Buy nonperishables in bulk when they're on sale.
- Use money-saving coupons.
- Obtain a benefits eligibility checklist from the local area agency on aging.
- Ask for discounts, especially when paying in full with cash on expensive items.
- Take advantage of senior citizen and group discounts.
- Use 800 toll-free telephone numbers whenever possible.
- Give gifts of time and personal service. Swap skills with others.
- Keep one car, sell the other.
- Look into less expensive housing options.
- Buy clothes that don't require dry cleaning.
- Ask a family member to help manage bill paying and spending.
- Get professional counseling in cases of gambling and credit card abuse.
- Ask a tax advisor about long-range financial and tax strategies.
- Eat meals at home—restaurants are relatively more expensive.
- Limit impulse buying—shop with a list and stick to it.
- Check loans, mortgages, and insurance policies for payment waivers.
- Repair air and water leaks.
- Check all bills for errors and overcharges.
- Make phone calls after the rates go down—or better yet, write.

PLAN THREE
Help reduce your elder's medical costs.

To cut the costs associated with health care, initiate conversations which include the following suggestions:

- Eat, drink, and exercise wisely.
- Manage medications.

• Get yearly medical and dental checkups.

• Instead of a doctor's office visit, discuss minor ailments over the telephone.

• Avoid hospital emergency rooms for nonemergencies. Locate a twenty-four-hour clinic.

• Consider group health insurance.

• Review health insurance policy for proper procedures *before* receiving treatment.

• Discuss *all* costs with doctor.

• Ask if tests in the doctor's office can be performed without a full office visit charge.

• Bring copies of medical records to every doctor's office visit.

• Get routine tests done before checking into the hospital.

• Fill prescriptions at the pharmacy rather than at the hospital pharmacy.

• Check out of the hospital before the checkout hour.

• Keep notes on doctor hospital visits and medications. Insist on itemized doctor and hospital bills. Review bills and insurance claims for errors.

• Preapprove the costs of hospital medical treatment and equipment.

• File all medical claims.

• Review continuation of medical insurance coverage for spouse upon elder's death.

PLAN FOUR
Review insurance policies to uncover room for savings.

To qualify for insurance deductions is well worth taking the time to review your elder's insurance papers. If the policy is not at hand, pick up the phone and call the insurance agent directly. Ask about the following discounts:

Multiple policy discounts may be offered to customers who agree to two or more policies with the same company.

Smoke and burglar alarm discounts for home and office. Ask about security device discounts on dead-bolt locks and special window locks.

Antitheft, automatic seat belts, airbags, antilock brakes, and low yearly mileage may also qualify for automobile discounts.

Nonsmoker discounts offered to home and auto policy holders. Also look into multicar discounts.

Fire-resistant discounts for homes and buildings made of special fire-proof materials. Rebates for attic insulation are also available.

Mature homeowner and driver discounts available for those over fifty-five years of age.

Long-term policy holder discounts are offered to those who keep a policy with the same company for several years. NOTE: Do not sign an insurance check until you're satisfied with the settlement.

PLAN FIVE
Discuss ways to reduce travel costs.

The cost of travel doesn't have to be expensive, especially for those who have flexible schedules. To reduce expenses, perhaps your relative will consider the following suggestions:

- Ask ahead about senior-citizen and group discounts.
- Travel midweek, off-season.
- Use 800 phone numbers to make reservations.
- Give consideration to travel cancellation insurance on expensive trips.
- Shop around for traveler's checks. Prices vary.
- Make friends with a travel agent who can notify you if someone cancels a trip at the last moment and then can resell the trip at a discount.
- Join a last-minute travel club.
- Check the reputation of all travel outfitters.
- Pack for emergencies: nonprescription painkillers, bandages, elastic bandages, thermometer, emergency sting kit, night light, flashlight, emergency telephone numbers, extra pair of prescription glasses, and an ample supply of prescription medicines.
- Stay at budget-priced motels.
- Know how to access emergency money if the need arises.
- Be a savvy shopper.

PLAN SIX
Consider the services of a financial advisor.

Financial advisors come in two categories: stockbrokers and financial planners. Stockbrokers are salespeople. They sell products like stocks, bonds, and tax-deferred annuities. Financial planners offer a broader perspective than stockbrokers. They look at your budget, savings, investments, insurance, and help to create short- and long-term financial goals. They are salespeople too, concentrating on mutual funds and annuities.

Anyone can call himself/herself a financial planner, so look for someone with a Certified Financial Planner (CFP) designation. Be cautious of a planner who makes recommendations before thoroughly reviewing your elder's financial goals. Additionally, financial planners must be registered with the Securities and Exchange Commission to make investment suggestions. If your elder's financial planner offers securities investment advice as part of his/her services and is not registered to do so, seek financial advice elsewhere. Ask prospective planners to provide past and current client references and to see their credentials.

No matter what your elder's age or tax bracket, there are financial plans that can save money on taxes. Some of the tax laws are complicated and it could take months to put strategies in place. Find a financial advisor who specializes in tax management.

Create short- and long-term financial plans with the help of a tax attorney, a certified public accountant, or a certified financial planner. Like most professional advisors, financial planners are best found through recommendations of trusted sources.

Interview prospective advisors by asking these questions:

How are your fees determined? (If hourly, get an estimate of the total.)
Is there a charge for the initial visit?
What are the ongoing costs of working with you?
Exactly what services are provided?
How much time is spent planning? consulting?
Are you available throughout the year or just during tax season?
Who will do the work? Accountant? Assistant?
How are clients kept informed of tax regulations?
Will you represent me if I'm called in for an audit?
Are you easily accessible?

PLAN SEVEN

Suggest building a cash reserve while increasing income.

Make the most out of your relative's present financial situation:

Hold a garage sale or call in an estate liquidator professional. The money realized from sales can be invested or used to pay bills. Liquidators are listed in the yellow pages under **Auctioneers, Junk Dealers, Second-Hand Dealers, Appraisers.**

Analyze investment income. In the quest for financial security, aging people tend to keep assets in low-yielding passbook savings. The following investment options show various risk ranges. A and B are lower risks than C and D. NOTE: Invest in the following options only through reputable investment dealers. Do not sign anything without reviewing options with a trusted advisor.

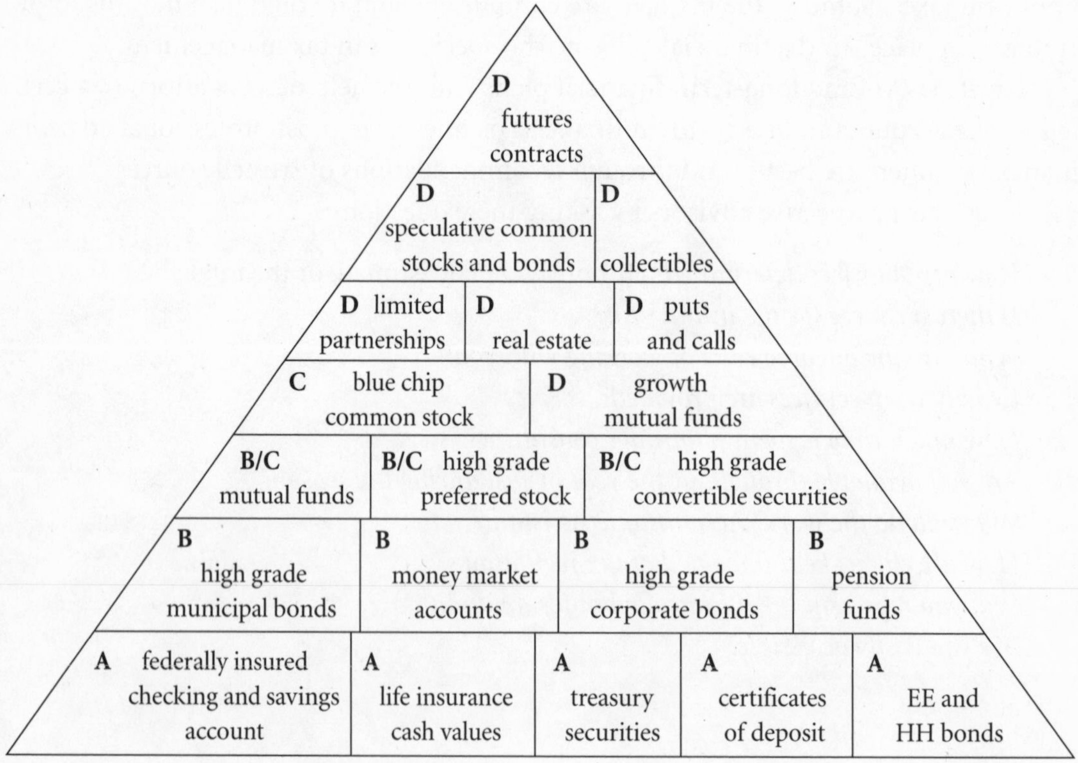
D futures contracts
D speculative common stocks and bonds
D collectibles
D limited partnerships
D real estate
D puts and calls
C blue chip common stock
D growth mutual funds
B/C mutual funds
B/C high grade preferred stock
B/C high grade convertible securities
B high grade municipal bonds
B money market accounts
B high grade corporate bonds
B pension funds
A federally insured checking and savings account
A life insurance cash values
A treasury securities
A certificates of deposit
A EE and HH bonds

PLAN EIGHT
Explore additional sources of retirement benefits, rebates, and reductions.

Tap into financial resources that are set aside specifically to help the elderly:

Social Security is a federal income program offered to individuals upon retirement age or upon becoming disabled. Social Security laws move the eligibility for full retirement benefits up to sixty-six years of age starting in the year 2005. At this printing, elders are eligible for Social Security benefits at the age of sixty-five. The laws governing Social Security eligibility change from time to time and could mean extra income. Benefits should be reviewed at least every three years since that is the maximum time allowed for benefit amounts to be contested. Apply for Social Security by telephone or by going to the local Social Security office.

General relief is allocated to elders of very low income who are not eligible for federally funded assistance. General relief may be obtained from the Department of Social and Health Services.

Benefits eligibility checklists are available through the local office of the area agency on aging and the Department of Social and Health Services. Some of the services available from the checklist include: adult day care, adult education, community care, consumer fraud and protection, property tax assistance, denture referral programs, driver's license discount, elder abuse protection, emergency assistance, food stamps, home-delivered meals and nutrition sites, housing, utility bills assistance, Medicaid, Medicare, ombudsman program, pharmaceutical service, Social Security, supplemental insurance, travel and tourism, and volunteer programs.

Veterans' benefits and pensions are available for eligible veterans and their dependents. Call the local Veterans Administration office.

Supplemental Security Income (SSI) provides monthly benefits to those with very low income, the aged, and persons with disabilities. SSI is available through the Social Security office. If your elder cannot visit the office, ask for a home visit.

Elders aged sixty-two and older with disabilities may qualify for tax postponement, homeowner's assistance, and renter's assistance. Contact the state tax office.

Grandparents raising grandchildren may qualify for Aid to Families with Dependent Children. Contact the Department of Social and Health Services.

Other state and community programs offer tax breaks, utility payment assistance, rent relief, public transportation fare decreases, and taxi coupons. Workers' unions and fraternal organizations may also offer benefits.

PLAN NINE
Accumulate cash through life insurance.

Whole life insurance is a policy that builds cash value while offering a death benefit. Some companies may pay a portion of the death benefit while the policy holder is still alive. To collect early, a doctor's statement may be needed that states the policy holder has less than six months to live.

Terminally ill patients may also choose to sell their life insurance policies to outside companies, known as **viatical settlement companies.** In return for naming the viatical company as the sole beneficiary, the sick client gets paid up to 85 percent of the policy's face value. When the patient dies, the viatical company collects on the policy. There are tax questions to address so consult a tax advisor.

PLAN TEN
Retrieve cash through the benefits of owning a house.

Implementing any one of the following financial strategies may be all that is necessary to keep your elder financially independent:

If your house-rich, cash-poor elder is willing to move, trading down to a smaller place may be a smart strategy. A one-time exclusion that exempts from taxes some of the capital gain from the house sale is available to individuals fifty-five years or older and if they lived in the house for at least three of the past five years.

If moving is not an option and the house appeals to you as an investment, you could buy the home and lease it back to your relative. The property becomes a source of income for the seller (elder) and gives the buyer (you) the tax advantages of rental property. Another option allows an outside investor to buy the home on a sale/leaseback or life tenancy legalized agreement.

If you have neither the money nor the desire to buy your family member's home and the mortgage is paid, a reverse mortgage allows residents to occupy the home while receiving income. The homeowner borrows against the value of the home and receives monthly or line-of-credit payments from a mortgage lender. The lender charges interest on the payments. No repayment of the interest or principal is required unless the home is sold or is no longer occupied by owner. NOTE: Reverse mortgages do not assure homeowners lifelong income or the right to remain in the home. Be fully informed.

A deferred payment loan from the government can be provided to low-income persons at a low-interest rate. The loan permits homeowners to defer payments of all principal interest until the homeowner dies or when the house is sold.

Homeowner equity accounts are offered by brokerage firms and banks that allow homeowners to set up a line of credit secured by the value of the home. Terms vary as do interest rates. Shop around.

Your relative may choose to give his/her home to a person or an institution. The gift recipient then agrees to pay the homeowner a set monthly or yearly income as long as he/she is alive.

PLAN ELEVEN
Give money directly.

Gifts of money to aging relatives can help make ends meet as well as enhance his/her quality of life. Family members might want to open an interest-bearing checking account for the purpose of paying for:

Transportation	Telephone calls
Groceries	House maintenance
Cable TV service	Travel
Clothes	Personal care
Lawn care	Home decorating
House renovating	Health care
Appliances/Furniture	Laundry/cleaners

PLAN TWELVE
Avoid unwelcome emotional complications when giving your elder cash directly.

Even under the worst of financial conditions, our aging family members can, at times, be too proud to accept money from anyone. Creating formalized agreements can make such transactions go smoothly.

Consider a split-interest purchase. Under this joint purchase agreement, you and your relative divide the cost of an investment and agree that he/she gets all of the income while living. You receive the assets and any capital gain after your elder dies.

Give your relative a loan. Legalize the agreement and mention the loan in your elder's will. After your relative dies, the money can be repaid from the estate, probably when the assets are sold.

Generous gifts and services can take the place of money:

New winter coat	Airline tickets
Postage stamps	Gift certificates
House cleaning services	Prepaid phone cards
Convenience items	Grocery items
Restaurant gift certificates	House maintenance
Cable TV service	Personal care services
Lawn care	Home decorating
House renovating	Household appliances
Club memberships	Magazine subscriptions
Entertainment	Furniture

PLAN THIRTEEN
Your relative might want to take on a part-time job.

Employment opportunities are not limited by experience or age. Many businesses welcome older people as employees. See Chapter Twelve, Quality of Life, page 207, for numerous job suggestions. NOTE: Working status may affect your elder's Social Security benefits. Regulations should be reviewed before taking any job.

PLAN FOURTEEN
Know the medicaid spending policies.

Review the state Medicaid spending policies to protect the assets of one spouse should the other go into a nursing facility. If this information is not sought ahead of time, over-spending can leave the remaining spouse virtually penniless and family members may be penalized for implementing certain spending strategies. Seek valuable advice from an elder law attorney.

Low Cost/Free Resources

The securities industry maintains a **Central Registration Depository (CRD)** about stock-brokers and their firms. A full report, usually free, is available from your state securities agency. Call the North American Securities Administration, (202) 737-0900, for the tele-phone number of your securities agency.

If financial planners give investment advice, they should be registered with the **Securities and Exchange Commission** in order to file an ADV report. If a planner does not have an ADV, he or she should not be advising your elder.

Family members may be eligible for **dependent-care tax breaks** if their aging relative lives with them. Seek the advice of a tax advisor.

Elders in danger of having home utilities turned off because of not paying bills can call the **utility company** to work out a payment plan.

The **telephone company** offers discounts and free-of-charge services to customers with hearing and sight disabilities. Contact the Special Needs Center of the telephone company.

AARP's Tax Aide Program and **VITA (Volunteer Income Tax Assistance)** offer tax ser-vices. Contact the IRS office. Services to homebound elderly are available.

The **IRS** offers Tele-Tax, an automated information line that offers recorded tax-topic in-formation.

Taxpayers' Rights Advocates can be found at the state board of equalization office.

Free medications. Some drug companies give people who can't afford their medications their drugs free of charge. Eligibility requirements vary. If your family member is eligible, the drug company sends the medications to the doctor for distribution. To obtain a list of participating drug companies call the Pharmaceutical Research and Manufacturers of America at (800)762-4636.

If you believe that cash and valuables have been forgotten about in bank accounts or a safe-deposit box, call the **state treasurer's office,** which keeps a list of unclaimed money and property.

Call the local office of the **Veterans Administration** to ask about eligibility benefits.

Catholic Charities provides nondenominational family and individual assistance with debt obligations. Loans and grants are available for qualified individuals.

ORGANIZATIONS

American Institute of Certified Public Accountants
1211 Avenue of the Americas, New York, NY 10036, (800) 862-4272,
(212) 596-6200

Consumer Information Center
Website *http://www.pueblo.gsa.gov*

Health Care Financing Administration (Medicare and Medicaid)
Website *http://www.hcfa.gov*

Institute of Certified Financial Planners
7600 E. Eastman Ave., Suite 301, Denver, CO 80231, (800) 282-7526,
(303) 751-7600

International Association for Financial Planning
5775 Glenridge Dr., NE, Suite B-300, Atlanta, GA 30328, (800) 945-4237
Website *http://www.iafp.org*

National Association of Personal Financial Advisors
1130 W. Lake Cook Road, Suite 150, Buffalo Grove, IL 60089, (800) 366-2732,
(888) 333-6659, (847) 577-7722

National Center for Home Equity Conversion
7373 147th St., West, Suite 115, Apple Valley, MN 55124, (612) 953-4474

National Committee to Preserve Social Security and Medicare
2000 K St., NW, Suite 800, Washington, DC 20006, (202) 822-9459,
(800) 966-1935

National Organization of Social Security Claimant's Representatives
9 E. Central Ave., Pearl River, NY 10965, (914) 735-8812, (800) 431-2804

Pension Rights Center
918 16th St., NW, Suite 704, Washington, DC 20006, (202) 296-3776

Medicare Hotline
(800) 638-6833

Social Security Administration
6401 Security Blvd., Room 4J5, Baltimore, MD 21235, (800) 772-1213
Website *http://www.ssa.gov*

The Wealth Center
Website *http://www.aecnet.com/matters*

Action Checklist

THE COST OF CARING	To Do By	Completed

Become familiar with eldercare-related expenses
(Plan One) . . .

elder's home	_____	❏
household items	_____	❏
basic living	_____	❏
home health care	_____	❏

Consider the cost of long-distance assistance . . .

travel	_____	❏
home	_____	❏
destination	_____	❏

Review your finances (Plan Two) . . .

keep written record	_____	❏
locate important documents	_____	❏

Consider ability to contribute to expenses (Plan Two). _____ ❏

Budget eldercare expenses (Plan Two) . . .

short-term	_____	❏
long-term	_____	❏

Protect personal financial stability (Plan Three). _____ ❏

Review elder's financial stability (Plan Four). _____ ❏

Develop a family plan (Plan Four) . . .

current expenses	_____	❏
future expenses	_____	❏

Create eldercare account (Plan Four) . . .

savings	_____	❏
checking account	_____	❏

Record and file eldercare expenses receipts (Plan Four). _____ ❏

Evaluate elder's financial needs every six months.   _____   ❏

Ask family to give time and resources (Plan Four).   _____   ❏

READY CASH

Set financial goals . . .
   short-term   _____   ❏
   long-term   _____   ❏

Complete cash flow analysis (Plan One).   _____   ❏

Reduce elder's . . .
   debts (Plan Two)   _____   ❏
   living expenses (Plan Two)   _____   ❏
   medical costs (Plan Three)   _____   ❏
   insurance costs (Plan Four)   _____   ❏
   travel expenses (Plan Five)   _____   ❏
   taxes (Plan Six)   _____   ❏

Increase elder's income . . .
   liquidation (Plan Seven)   _____
   investments (Plan Seven)   _____   ❏
   Social Security (Plan Eight)   _____   ❏
   veteran's benefits (Plan Eight)   _____   ❏
   pensions (Plan Eight)   _____   ❏
   relief programs (Plan Eight)   _____   ❏
   life insurance (Plan Nine)   _____   ❏
   home ownership (Plan Ten)   _____   ❏
   gifts/loans (Plans Eleven, Twelve)   _____   ❏
   employment (Plan Thirteen)   _____   ❏

Learn the state Medicaid spending policy (Plan Fourteen).   _____   ❏

Plan for elder's . . .
   housing expenses   _____   ❏
   living expenses   _____   ❏
   medical expenses   _____   ❏

READY CASH	To Do By	Completed
insurance	_____	❑
service providers	_____	❑
funeral expenses	_____	❑

Record the phone number of elder's . . .

tax accountant	_____	❑
legal advisor	_____	❑
bank	_____	❑
financial advisor	_____	❑
insurance agents	_____	❑

Keep phone numbers . . .

at home	_____	❑
at work	_____	❑
in wallet/purse	_____	❑

Distribute phone numbers to key people.   _____   ❑

Chapter 5

LEGAL MATTERS

Estate Planning

There are many advantages to estate planning but some people choose not to plan their estates. Why? Several reasons: They may not know of the option; they don't want to spend their money on attorney's fees; they simply find it hard to discuss and make decisions for what occurs after their death.

Most of us are not wealthy and have limited assets. Therefore we may not see the value of addressing estate-planning issues. The most popular argument for avoiding such matters is that most people assume their affairs are legally in order because they own everything jointly with their heirs. *This can be a costly mistake.*

As a way to take action, ask yourself what might happen to *your* financial future if your relative lives longer than expected. In addition to planning for what happens to family assets in the event of death, the foundation of estate planning also includes the preservation and distribution of "wealth" before death. In an age where people are living one third longer than they thought they would, it is wise to investigate options now.

This section of the planner simplifies the process of estate planning. You will gain a basic understanding of the legal terms and how proper planning provides for orderly distribution of assets while minimizing court delays, fees, and taxes. This way, gifts, title transfer, contracts, and trusts can be coordinated to maximize the financial benefits.

ESTATE PLANNING

- Without a will the state will divide property with no regard for the family's special needs. The state will select heirs, leave unnecessarily large bequests to the tax collector, and will charge for services.
- Estate planning not only focuses on property distribution after death, but also on protecting hard-earned assets during an elder's lifetime.
- If people fail to plan in advance for incapacity, the state has the authority to set standards as to what the incompetent patient would want.

If your aging family member is avoiding estate planning, perhaps taking the process step-by-step and locating affordable, easy-to-understand assistance will spare everyone unnecessary expenses and anguish.

Objectives

After completing Estate Planning you will be able to:

Gain basic knowledge of estate planning terms and legal forms.

Locate affordable elder law resources.

Maintain control of decisions in the event of your elder's incapacity.

Avoid the devastating consequences of the absence of legal documentation.

Get to know the basic estate-planning terms and options.

Estate-planning terms are easier to understand when you approach them step-by-step:

A **will** describes how an individual wants his/her estate to be distributed upon death. The document may include provisions for a trust and usually names an executor. Wills need to be updated because of change of mind, change of inheritance, assets not covered in previous will, marriage, birth, death, adoption, divorce, and new laws mandating changes.

Trustee/Executor are individuals designated by the creator of the will who will see to it that the will is properly executed. A trustee manages a trust and an executor sees that specific provisions of the will are followed, pays estate taxes, debits, and expenses. The trustee and executor can be the same person.

Trust is a way to leave money that takes advantage of tax benefits and accomplishes the desires of the person setting up the trust. A trust controls the release of money before or after death. There are dozens of different types of trusts.

Living trust transfers stocks, property, and other items from one living person to another, avoids probate, and also protects in the event of incapacity. A revocable living trust gives the creator of the trust the right to change the terms of the trust or even end it. Living trusts do not save taxes as compared to a will.

Testamentary trust assures that all assets to beneficiaries are received upon the death of the creator of the trust. This trust can be designed to end after a specified period of time, before or after the person's death. After the death of the testator, this trust becomes an irrevocable trust.

Letter of instruction is prepared for the beneficiaries of the will and trust. The letter is meant to serve as a guide for closing out the life affairs of an individual upon his/her death. Although this letter is not a legal document, the composition should be in agreement with the individual's will. The letter of instruction should also include people to notify when death occurs, disposal of possessions, and funeral desires.

Durable power of attorney gives a person legal right to sign his/her name to business transacted in another person's name. This power must be arranged while the individual is still competent, and can be terminated at any time upon the person's written request. NOTE: Banks and other financial institutions typically do not honor power of attorney forms other than their own. Check with each banking institution to obtain proper documents. Be aware that some states order safe-deposit boxes sealed upon the tenant's death and they are not opened until a state tax commission representative is present. Other states require a court order to open a box rented in the decedent's sole name.

PLAN TWO
Seek legal advice.

Family members should resist the temptation to draft their own will. Nonlegalized documents might be contested in court or heirs may end up paying more estate taxes than they should.

A simple will can cost as little as a few hundred dollars. Keep original copies of legal documents in a safe, twenty-four-hour accessible place, leaving copies of the documents with the attorney. Remind your relative to keep the contents of legal documents up-to-date.

Locating the services of an estate-planning attorney can be accomplished through personal referrals, attorney referrals services, or by calling the local bar association. Check the attorney's qualifications and shop around to compare fees, services, and experience.

PLAN THREE
Simplify the will by giving things away ahead of time.

Money and property are not the only assets your aging family member may have. There are clothes, household supplies, furniture, photographs, books, letters, collections, jewels, and other items. Some people prefer to dispose of personal possessions and mementos as they age, enjoying the giving process as they go. Others prefer distributing personal possessions through a letter of instruction as part of their will.

PLAN FOUR
Plan for incapacity to maintain control over your elder's affairs.

Few people plan for disability or incapacity. The result is often a loss of control over who will make decisions. Proper planning will allow financial and health care considerations to be made without court intervention or conservatorship proceedings. Consider the following methods:

> **Durable power of attorney** is legal documentation transferring the power of decision making to a designated person and continues to give power of attorney in the event of incapacity. This document must be completed while your relative is still competent. Regular powers of attorney are not honored in these situations.

> **Durable power of attorney for health care** gives another person legal authority to make medical decisions in the event of incapacity. Aging family members can specify how these decisions are to be made and must be of informed consent and sound mind when implementing this document. It is not necessary to hire an attorney to complete this document. Request a durable power of attorney for health care form from the hospital social services director. Have the completed forms reviewed for accuracy by a qualified social worker employed by the hospital. Services are provided on a sliding fee scale or they are provided free of charge. Otherwise see an attorney to complete this document.

> **Legal guardian/Conservatorship** is a legal process for assuming control over an already incapacitated individual's affairs. This is usually the last method considered. A court hearing is required.

> **Directives to physician** instructs a doctor to withhold medical treatment if it would not aid in recovery, only prolong death. If the doctor disagrees ahead of time with any key terms, consider switching physicians. Include these instructions in the durable power of attorney for health care document. Instruction also should be left by those who do not want their lives ended by the withdrawal of treatment, no matter how ill or long they are incapacitated. Forms are available at doctors' offices and retirement and nursing homes.

> **Living will** is a document that states the medical situations under which patients would not want to be kept alive. Some doctors and hospitals may refuse to honor

this document. State laws vary widely. NOTE: The medical system is set up to save lives and is reluctant to turn away a dying patient, no matter what the wishes of that individual. A living will holds many limitations and is not legally binding. This is why the durable power of attorney for health care is a more binding document.

PLAN FIVE
Make estate planning instructions known.

Legalized forms, documents, and instructions don't do a bit of good unless family members are made aware of their existence. Be sure that your relative has distributed and discussed the contents of important information with designated family members, doctors, friends, nursing home facility directors, and all others. NOTE: Keep original documents in a safe-deposit box or in a safe, twenty-four-hour accessible place, giving lawyers copies instead of originals. You or your elder may want to switch attorneys later on.

Family members should carry notice of his/her durable power of attorney for health care at all times. Elder's designated agents should be prepared to present proof of this document at a moment's notice.

If a relative enters the hospital or a nursing home facility, attach copies of any directives to his/her medical charts. Ask nursing home directors to agree, in writing, to comply with your elder's wishes.

Remind family members to update all documentation as needed.

Elder Advocacy

In less than three years, the United States Census Bureau estimates that our elderly population over the age of eighty-five will be triple what it is today. With this kind of growth in an aging population, the well-being of government social service and health care programs serving the elderly is in serious financial jeopardy. Every year, policy makers cut the budgets and staff of these organizations, placing practically the entire burden of eldercare on the backs of family, friends, and volunteers.

The current lack of easily accessible eldercare programs already makes the family caregiver's task an endurance test. Family members are often overwhelmed by the red tape of their fact-finding mission. Time and stamina quickly wear thin. To make matters worse, most elderly Americans do not meet the rigid criteria to qualify for the government's free and low-cost services. Programs like Medicare do not pay for the basic day-to-day care and assistance that most elderly people require.

This section of the planner encourages you and your family members to become active advocates for improvements in eldercare social services. Get involved and join the fight for the right to keep eldercare programs alive.

ELDER ADVOCACY

- Be aware that some policy makers want to turn back the clock and place practically the entire burden of eldercare on the backs of family, friends, and volunteers.
- There is a critical need for programs that help families take care of aging relatives as well as programs that help relatives help themselves.
- Overt acts of discrimination are an everyday concern for older people.

One of the most effective ways to safeguard the well-being of the elderly is to protect the rights of senior citizens and join in the fight for responsible government policies.

Objectives

*After completing **Elder Advocacy** you will be able to:*

Keep in contact with politicians who are responsible for eldercare policies.

Stay involved and informed with policies affecting elderly Americans.

PLAN ONE
Keep an alert and wary eye on politicians.

Monitor the activities of politicians who consider programs for elderly Americans an expense, not an investment:

- Stay informed.
- Attend local government meetings.
- Vote.

PLAN TWO
Protect the present and the future of the elderly by getting involved.

Local, state, and federal eldercare programs exist as a result of various activities of advocacy groups. Become a member. Lobbyists will notify you when the time is right for sending letters to legislators. Letters add up to action and when election time rolls around, politicians need the seniors' votes. Political action takes dedication and energy. Join others in making important changes in eldercare policies and services, locally and nationwide.

PLAN THREE
Fight for improved eldercare policies and programs.

Topics of elder advocacy that deserve attention are . . .

Health care	Long-term care
Home health care	Nursing home policies
Social Security	Medicare
Supplemental health insurance	Medicaid
Senior community activity programs	Tax programs
Elder law	Nutrition programs
Transportation services	Employment and job training
Education	Senior centers funding
Pension entitlements	Subsidized housing
Retirement policies	Estate planning
Funeral arrangement policies	Disability policies

Contact the following advocates if you suspect that any elderly person's rights are being violated: long-term care ombudsman, social workers, family counselors, family service agencies, hospital social services director, area agency on aging, AARP, Gray Panthers, and the department of social services' adult protection services.

Low Cost/Free Resources

Legal advice is available for elders with limited incomes. Contact the area agency on aging, the local bar association, AARP, or the district attorney's office. You might also call a local law school to find out if it offers a legal clinic serving the community.

The **secretary of state's office** has a TDD (telecommunications device for the deaf) for voter registration and election information. For persons with visual disabilities, audio tapes of the state and county candidates are available in the county clerk–recorder's office.

If you wish to reach your **senator** or **representative**, write directly. Address envelope to: Senator (Name), U.S. Senate, Washington, DC 20510 or Representative (Name), U.S. House of Representatives, Washington, DC 20515. The Capitol hotline is (800) 972-3524.

Free copies of the **durable power of attorney for health care** forms are available at your local area agency on aging and the hospital social services department. Many hospitals provide free advice for filling out these forms.

ORGANIZATIONS

American Bar Association
750 N. Lake Shore Drive, Chicago, IL 60611, (800) 285-2221, (312) 988-5000
Website *http://www.abanet.org*

Close Up Program for Older Americans
44 Canal Center Plaza, Alexandria, VA 22314, (800) 232-2000

Legal Counsel for the Elderly (AARP)
PO Box 96474, Washington, DC 20090, (202) 434-2174

The Long Term Care Campaign
PO Box 27394, Washington, DC 20038, (202) 434-3744
E-mail: *hn6533@handsnet.org*

National Academy of Elder Law Attorneys
1604 N. Country Club Road, Tucson, AZ 85716, (520) 881-4005
Website *http://www.naela.com/elderlaw*

National Association for Hispanic Elderly
3325 Wilshire Blvd., Suite 800, Los Angeles, CA 90010, (213) 487-1784

National Caucus and Center on the Black Aged
1424 K St., NW, Suite 500, Washington, DC 20005, (202) 637-8400

National Clearinghouse for Legal Services
205 W. Monroe, Second Floor, Chicago, IL 60606, (312) 263-3830

National Council of Senior Citizens
Department of Public Affairs and Legislation, 1331 F St., NW, Washington, DC 20004, (202) 624-9535, (202) 624-9539

National Hispanic Council on Aging
2713 Ontario Road, NW, Suite 200, Washington, DC 20009, (202) 265-1288

National Indian Council on Aging
6400 Uptown Blvd., NE, City Center, Suite 510-W, Albuquerque, NM 87110, (505) 888-3302

National Pacific/Asian Resource Center on Aging
Melbourne Tower, 1511 3rd Street, Suite 914, Seattle, WA 98101, (206) 624-1221

National Senior Citizen Law Center
1815 H St., NW, Suite 700, Washington, DC 20006, (202) 887-5280
Website *http://www.nscla.org*

Older Women's League
666 11th St., NW, Suite 700, Washington, DC 20001, (202) 783-6686

Action Checklist

ESTATE PLANNING	To Do By	Completed
Set estate-planning goals . . .		
short-term	_____	❏
long-term	_____	❏
Locate elder-law resources (Plan Two).	_____	❏
Draw up (Plans One, Four) . . .		
will	_____	❏
trust	_____	❏
letter of instruction	_____	❏
durable power of attorney	_____	❏
durable power of attorney for health care	_____	❏
Duplicate, distribute, and review documents with key family members.	_____	❏
Store original documents (Plan Five).	_____	❏
Plan to review and update legal documents.	_____	❏
Keep a notice of durable power of attorney . . .		
at home	_____	❏
at work	_____	❏
in wallet/purse	_____	❏
Obtain important phone numbers.	_____	❏
Keep copies of phone numbers . . .		
at home	_____	❏
at work	_____	❏
in wallet/purse	_____	❏
Distribute phone numbers to key people.	_____	❏
Read information on estate planning.	_____	❏

ELDER ADVOCACY

Join senior citizen advocacy groups . . .

AARP ☐

Gray Panthers ☐

Older Women's League ☐

other ☐

Know how to reach . . .

city hall ☐

village office ☐

mayor's office ☐

city council members ☐

U.S. senator ☐

U.S. representative ☐

governor's office ☐

Vote . . .

local elections ☐

national elections ☐

Stay informed. Read . . .

community newspapers ☐

city newspapers ☐

political flyers ☐

Chapter 6

INSURANCE

Insurance Coverage for a Longer Life

We cannot live our lives as if a crisis is about to occur. We can, however, plan so that if something does happen, proper insurance coverage can minimize its effects on the entire family. Taking the time now to insure for a longer life will help family caregivers and their relatives feel more secure in the long run.

A review of existing insurance policies will reveal under and over insurance coverage. It also may disclose the absence of insurance coverage that should be in place. Insurance needs may have changed since the purchase of the policy and now, rather than under emergency conditions, is the time to gather and review your elder's insurance documents.

This section of the planner will help you familiarize yourself with your elder's insurance coverage. Establishing a relationship with his/her insurance agent and asking for explanations on policy coverage and limitations will help eliminate potential insurance problems. Have the agent explain all details so you can fully understand the policy and are satisfied with its provisions.

INSURANCE COVERAGE FOR A LONGER LIFE

- Insurance is often one service purchased without adequate information.
- Insurance needs may have changed since the purchase of the policy.

If it has been more than one year since your elder's insurance policies have been reviewed, now would be a good time to check for too much or too little protection.

Objectives

*After completing **Insurance Coverage for a Longer Life** you will be able to:*

Know if insurance coverage has been secured.

Bring insurance coverage up to date.

Examine an insurance company's financial stability.

PLAN ONE

Scrutinize your relative's insurance policies for overcoverage and undercoverage.

Review the conditions under which the policies were purchased for homeowner, auto, life insurance, disability, personal property, and business insurance. Renewing present insurance policies for adequate coverage may be less expensive than purchasing additional insurance. Note any changes in beneficiaries.

The most important role of insurance is to protect from catastrophe. The cost of insurance depends on the rate of the deductible. Extended personal-liability insurance (umbrella coverage) can be coordinated with the family member's home and auto insurance.

Insurance is big business and insurance agents make money selling insurance policies. Television ads and mail offers with entertainers and political figures as spokespersons can be misleading. These people are paid to sell insurance and their image does not guarantee the quality of the policies advertised.

A reputable, licensed insurance agent, who comes referred from a trusted source, will be valuable in helping you investigate insurance options. The local department on aging will be able to offer family members the names of insurance advisors who advocate the special insurance needs of the elderly. Policies should be reviewed by a third party before signing on the dotted line.

Following are a few of the insurance plans you should know:

Homeowner—The amount of insurance to carry depends on the replacement value of the house or what it would cost to rebuild it as it now stands. Do not confuse this concept with market value. Make sure that replacement costs keep up with inflation.

Possessions—Blanket coverage under homeowner and renter's insurance policies is limited. Valuables should be itemized and insured individually.

Auto—To save money on premiums, take higher deductibles on automobile collision, fire, theft, or vandalism. If the vehicle is more than six years old, experts recommend dropping collision coverage altogether. The insurer will pay no more than car market value. Lost wage protection is unnecessary for nonworking elders, yet most are paying for it on their auto insurance policy.

Life insurance—Aging family members could carry life insurance if there are dependents who would suffer financially when they died. People also buy life insurance to pay for inheritance tax and probate costs, debts, mortgages, outstanding education bills, nursing home care, real estate, business, health care, and funeral expenses. Note any changes of beneficiaries.

Disability—Experts agree that anyone who has a job should consider a disability policy. Proper coverage averages 60 percent of a person's salary for as long as the policyholder cannot work. The policy should also state that it is noncancelable and renewable at the original premium until at least the age of sixty-five.

PLAN TWO
Take inventory.

Inventory lists or photographic inventory of your elder's household and business possessions are essential in establishing the proper amount of coverage needed. Videotaped records work just as well. Should there be reason to collect insurance benefits, photographs and videos will be of great value in obtaining a fair settlement. Keep photos and negatives separate. Store negatives in a safe-deposit box along with other important documentation.

If your family member needs to file a loss claim, the insurance agent will need a written report of the items. Videos can be used as a tool for memory recall, which is critical when making a claim.

Valuables should be itemized. The insurance company will require sales receipts and appraisals for all valuables. Keep receipts in a safe-deposit box.

PLAN THREE
Protect against unstable insurance investments.

If your elder's financial future depends on payments from an insurer, examine that company's stability. Insolvencies are likely to rise as a result of bad investments and some states do not guarantee funds when an insurer goes broke. Investors cannot count on warnings of impending insolvencies from regulators.

Know the insurer's rating by each of the following established companies: A. M. Best,

Moody's, Standard and Poor, and Duff and Phelps. If the insurance company is assessed by only one of these companies, that could indicate a problem. You will find these rate books at the public library.

Contact the insurer's home office and request the most recent quarterly and annual reports. Review the quality of the insurer's investments as these investments provide the income it needs to meet financial obligations to policyholders.

Beyond Medicare

Medicare, the government health insurance plan for older Americans, offers minimal coverage for health-care costs. Existing gaps in this basic insurance program mean your aging family members are unprotected from today's soaring health-care expenditures. A chronic illness such as arthritis or diabetes can put the financial resources of the entire family at serious risk since Medicare will not pay for the kind of day-to-day care these illnesses demand.

To help customers make informed health-care insurance decisions, Congress imposed tougher standards on supplemental insurers (also known as Medigap insurers). Companies are required to sell standardized policies so that customers can easily compare competitive products. To ease comparison procedures, insurers must also provide potential buyers with detailed outlines of policy coverage.

States across the country are in the process of setting up or expanding counseling programs on Medicare, Medicaid, and other health-care coverage issues. Encourage relatives to take advantage of this free advice to ensure a wise choice in their health insurance supplement.

This section of the planner stresses the importance of understanding the coverage and limitations of Medigap policies and the steps you can take to avoid insurance denial and policy cancellation.

BEYOND MEDICARE

- If medical bills are not at least partially covered by an employer's insurance plan and your relative does not carry a Medigap policy, the wealth of the family is at serious risk.
- Medicare benefits exclude chronically ill elders who need some form of long-term, nonskilled nursing care.
- The rule to buying supplemental health insurance is to review and compare policy differences. If what the insurance company offers sounds too good to be true, it is.

Since Medicare does not cover all of a patient's medical expenses, buying some form of health insurance supplement is essential.

Objectives

*After completing **Beyond Medicare** you will be able to:*

Distinguish Medicare from health insurance supplement policies.

Locate insurance advisors.

Review Medicare HMO options.

Protect against long-term-care insurance denial or policy cancellation.

PLAN ONE
Become familiar with health insurance options.

Health insurance plans for the elderly include:

Medicare is a federal insurance program that covers a portion of medical and hospital bills for those sixty-five years of age and older, regardless of income, and those already receiving Social Security benefits. The program is actually two health plans in one. Part A (hospital) and Part B (medical). Part B is not free and requires a monthly premium payment. Even if your relative is not on Social Security, he/she can elect to receive Medicare coverage. File for Medicare with the local Social Security office. If your elder disagrees with a Part A Medicare decision about what and how much is covered as well as the quality of the care, he/she can appeal to the organization that refused to pay the claim. Disagreements about Part B can be reviewed by the private insurer Medicare contracts to process claims. The appeal process for Part A is currently sixty days, and six months for Part B.

Medicaid is federal and state assistance that helps pay medical bills for low-income people of all ages.

Qualified Medicare Beneficiaries (QMB) and Specified Low-income Medicare Beneficiaries (SLMB) are part of the Medicaid program that is supposed to pay Medicare premiums, deductibles, and co-payments for low-income enrollees. Any state, welfare, social service, or public health agency that takes Medicaid applications also takes QMB and SLMB applications.

Medigap supplementary insurance bridges the gap between what Medicare pays for and what your elder must pay.

PLAN TWO
Explore the need for supplementary health insurance coverage.

Standardized Medigap supplemental insurance policies pay for some or all hospital deductibles and doctor co-payments not covered by Medicare. These policies must conform to one of ten standard plans designed to provide a specific range of benefits. Companies or agents are prohibited by law from selling your elder more than one Medigap policy. Seek information regarding optional benefits when traveling outside the United States.

If there is a chance that your elder may forget to pay premiums, arrange for automated bill paying and ask the insurance company to send you duplicates of the bills. Seek health insurance coverage through . . .

Group coverage—insurance policies obtained through job, club memberships, fraternal and religious groups, workers' unions, and the chamber of commerce.

Medicare Health Maintenance Organizations (HMOs), Preferred Provider Organizations (PPOs), and Individual Practice Associations (IPAs)—prepaid insurance plans based on preventive health care.

Private hospital policies—offered through local hospitals.

Private insurance companies—offer various coverage and payment plans.

PLAN THREE
Implement health insurance safeguards.

Knowing these basic insurance regulations keeps your elder's coverage in check . . .

- Buy only one supplement policy, get rid of duplicates. *(It's the law.)*
- If eligible for Medicaid, don't buy additional policies.
- If an employer offers retirees health insurance, consider taking it.
- Review continuation of medical insurance coverage for spouse upon elder's death.
- Waiting periods are not allowed when one Medigap policy is bought to replace another.
- The insurance company must offer coverage regardless of a person's medical history, for a six-month period after turning sixty-five years of age. Don't miss this deadline.

If your family member is considering the Medicare HMO option, ask the provider these questions . . .

What services are covered?
Is the plan accredited?
When I need to see the doctor, how long must I wait for an appointment?
If I am unsatisfied, how easy is it to switch primary-care physicians?

How many HMO members leave? Why do they leave?

What is the appeals process if payment for care is denied?

What prescription drugs are covered?

What are the reasons for care payment denial?

How do members get care while traveling outside of the HMO service area?

How do you accommodate members who move outside of the service area or spend part of each year away from home?

Will you provide a list of nursing homes and home health-care agencies? (The unavailability of a written list may mean that the HMO is reserving the right to wait and choose these services based on cost rather than the quality of care provided.)

PLAN FOUR
Know the Medicaid spending policies.

State Medicaid spending policies protect the assets of one spouse should the other go into a nursing facility. If professional advice is not sought ahead of time, overspending can leave the remaining spouse virtually penniless and family members may be penalized for implementing certain spending strategies. Seek valuable advice from an elder law attorney.

PLAN FIVE
Be aware that long-term-care insurance policies may be riddled with loopholes.

In order to capture their share of the market, insurance companies are developing policies that cover long-term care such as domestic help and personal-care services so that elderly people can remain in their own homes. However, there may be a big gap between what consumers think they bought and the kind of help they will actually receive. Many policies do not provide immediate at-home help and go into effect sixty to ninety days after a hospital stay. Also, strict criteria must be met before a policy covers assistance to someone who simply needs help with domestic chores and with eating, dressing, and bathing. The situation has to be far more serious than most people expect. NOTE: Insurance coverage or benefits may be denied if the company can prove fraudulent statements were made on the application. Also, the cost of the insurance may jump to nonaffordable levels forcing customers to drop the policy.

Follow these purchasing guidelines . . .

- Applicants, not insurance agents, fill out the medical questions on the application.
- Answer all questions truthfully and completely. If an agent says not to list a health condition, find another agent.
- During the free-look period (thirty days after the policy is delivered), check the application to make sure that the agent answered the questions correctly and has not changed your elder's answers. If an error is spotted, notify the company immediately and get the company's response in writing.
- Submit a physician's statement along with application. Demand written proof of acknowledgment from the insurance company that they have received this information and have filed it with your elder's insurance policy. Make a copy of the physician's statement and attach it to the insurance policy.
- Beware of agents who say they can get you coverage in a very short period of time (twenty-four to forty-eight hours).
- Beware of insurance companies that are willing to sell an insurance policy to anyone over the age of eighty-five.
- Check with the state insurance department to see if they have information on how the company in question pays claims or engages in "post-claims underwriting"—the practice of health insurance companies who check policyholders' medical history only after a claim is filed, instead of when the application is taken.
- Avoid policies that require hospitalization before a nursing home stay and those that require a prior level of care before benefits are payable.
- Look for policies that make no distinction between levels of care—skilled, custodial, and intermediate—and will pay for any type of care in any licensed facility. If the definitions seem too restrictive, look for another policy.
- A policy should cover respite care (to allow a family member a break) and adult day care.
- Buy one good policy, then upgrade to higher benefits or less-restrictive coverage. Upgrading may be less expensive than buying a new policy.
- If switching insurance companies, keep coverage on your old policy until receiving coverage on the new one.
- Make sure that the policy is guaranteed renewable and contains an inflation

rider. Understand the length of time or duration of coverage. Benefits should last at least three years.

• Look for an A or better rating in the A. M. Best Company book found at the public library.

• Avoid policies that do not specifically cover Alzheimer's and other dementia.

• Know that out-of-state group coverage is governed by laws of the state in which issued.

Low Cost/Free Resources

Refer to the telephone directory blue pages government section to locate **Government Insurance Assistance.**

The **State Insurance Commission** may be able to give information on the integrity of insurance companies and answer questions about a policy. Refer to the telephone directory blue pages government section under Insurance.

To obtain **Medicare** and **Medicaid** visit or call the Social Security office. Home visits from agency representatives also are available.

The local **area agency on aging** or **county office on aging** assists elders with Medicare billing problems and insurance policy selections. They also provide lists of participating health care providers.

A comprehensive **health insurance plan** is available through the State Insurance Commission. This is a government-sponsored program that helps people who have trouble getting insured. Refer to the telephone directory blue pages government section under **Insurance.**

Unbiased **health insurance counseling** is available by contacting the State Insurance Commission or getting referrals for advisors through the hospital discharge planner and the local area agency on aging.

ORGANIZATIONS

American Council of Life Insurance
1001 Pennsylvania Ave., NW, Washington, DC 20004, (202) 624-2000

Civilian Health and Medical Program of the Department of Veteran Affairs
CHAMP VA Center, PO Box 65023, Denver, CO 80222, (800) 733-8387

Health Care Financing Administration (Medicare and Medicaid)
Website *http://www.hcfa.gov*

Health Insurance Association of America
555 13th St., NW, Suite 600 East, Washington, DC 20004, (800) 635-1271

Insurance Information Institute
1750 K St., NW, Suite 1101, Washington, DC 20006, (202) 833-1580
Website *http://www.iii.org*

National Association of Insurance Commissioners
120 W. 12th St., Suite 1100, Kansas City, MO 64105, (816) 842-3600
Website *http://www.naic.org*

National Committee for Quality Assurance (to rate an HMO)
Website *http://www.ncqa.org*

Medicare Hotline
(800) 638-6833

National Committee to Preserve Social Security and Medicare
2000 K St., NW, Suite 800, Washington, DC 20006, (202) 822-9459

National Health Council
1730 M St., NW, Suite 500, Washington, DC 20036, (202) 785-3910

National Insurance Consumer Helpline
(800) 942-4242

Action Checklist

INSURANCE COVERAGE FOR A LONGER LIFE	To Do By	Completed

Review insurance policies for proper coverage (Plan One) . . .

homeowner	_____	❑
auto	_____	❑
life	_____	❑
disability	_____	❑
business	_____	❑
valuables	_____	❑

Set insurance coverage goals . . .

short-term	_____	❑
long-term	_____	❑

Review life insurance company for stability (Plan Three). _____ ❑

Locate a reputable, trusted insurance agent. _____ ❑

Review policies with insurance advisor. _____ ❑

Take inventory (Plan Two) . . .

photographs	_____	❑
inventory lists	_____	❑
video	_____	❑

Store inventory documents in a safe, twenty-four-hour accessible place. _____ ❑

Know phone numbers of elder's insurance agents. _____ ❑

Keep copies of phone numbers . . .

at home	_____	❑
at work	_____	❑
in wallet/purse	_____	❑

Give insurance phone numbers to key people. _____ ❑

Keep proof of insurance . . .

in car	_____	❑
in wallet/purse	_____	❑

BEYOND MEDICARE	To Do By	Completed
Apply for Medicare (Plan One) ...		
Part A	_____	❑
Part B	_____	❑
Research Medicaid spending policy (Plan Four).	_____	❑
Get a health insurance agent.	_____	❑
Shop and compare insurance options (Plan Two) ...		
group coverage	_____	❑
HMO	_____	❑
PPO	_____	❑
IPA	_____	❑
private hospital	_____	❑
private insurance company	_____	❑
Review for long-term care restrictions (Plan Five).	_____	❑
Know the phone numbers of ...		
Social Security office	_____	❑
supplementary insurance	_____	❑
Keep health insurance phone numbers ...		
at home	_____	❑
at work	_____	❑
in wallet/purse	_____	❑
Give health insurance phone numbers to key people.	_____	❑
Make copy of elder's health insurance card.	_____	❑
Stay informed ...		
Medicare	_____	❑
Medicaid	_____	❑
supplementary insurance	_____	❑
long-term-care insurance	_____	❑
Monitor elder's health insurance claims.	_____	❑

Chapter 7

HOUSING

Home Suite Home

Inevitable transitions in an aging person's lifestyle—retirement, chronic illness, repositioning of finances, and limited mobility—signal that it is time for the entire family to examine their elder's housing needs. The fact that our aging family member may have to
live elsewhere now or in the future means we have to make great adjustments.

Contrary to popular belief, most of the elderly are not ill. Only 6 percent of people
over the age of sixty-five require skilled nursing home care. The majority of the aging population live independently—even with their "aches and pains"—with the help of family,
friends, and assisted-living community programs. Study after study indicates that most
elderly people want to remain in their own homes and communities, but lack of proper
planning often forces them to live otherwise. Moving, and even remodeling, is a traumatic
experience for anyone. Minimize the negative reactions to changes in a living environment
by proceeding thoroughly and slowly, especially if your relative recently has experienced
a major loss or other serious stress.

To assume that nursing home care and having your aging family member move in
with you are the only options is outdated thinking. Unless your elder requires twenty-four-
hour supervision and extensive health care assistance, there are other choices available for
alternate, less expensive housing and care.

On the other hand, family caregivers may be reluctant to consider the nursing home
option when they should. The time may come when we can't do it all or don't have the
resources to give our aging relative the proper care required. Yes, the decision to place an
elder in a nursing home is a difficult one, but sometimes it is the only alternative. It is not
a question of whether or not institutionalized care is inherently good or bad. The decision for this option should be based on health-care needs, preference of the family care-

giver, finances, and the availability of quality facilities. The choice is very personal and can be a major life transition for the entire family.

During these times, open communication and planning ahead are vital. This section of the planner will guide you through the maze of investigating housing and care options while emphasizing the importance of making decisions that work to the benefit of the entire family.

HOME SUITE HOME

- Contrary to popular belief, most older people are not ill. Only 6 percent of those over sixty-five occupy some kind of nursing-care institution.
- 86 percent of Americans who are sixty or older have no desire to change their housing, but a lack of planning may force them to do so.
- With adequate information and planning, aging people can control their housing destinies. Polls indicate 88 percent of family members never discuss their housing needs with anyone.

If living arrangements do not meet your aging family member's lifestyle needs now and for the future, proactive planning could prevent last-minute, regrettable housing decisions.

Objectives

After completing Home Suite Home you will be able to:

Evaluate your relative's current and future lifestyle needs.

Recognize housing circumstances that may require immediate attention.

Locate alternate housing resources.

Find opportunities to get on waiting lists for housing options.

Minimize the trauma of moving.

Take a family consensus before your aging relative moves in.

PLAN ONE
**Be aware of circumstances that may determine a change in
your elder's housing.**

Consider the following circumstances that could change your aging family member's
housing status:

Finances	Little social activity
Home maintenance	Need for recreation
Demanding house chores	Lack of companionship
Lifestyle	Safety/Security
Climate	Stairs
Access to:	Isolation
Family/Caregivers/Friends	Lack of privacy
Medical care	Space
Transportation	Delivery routes
Shopping	Familiar surroundings
Place of worship	Memories
Family history	Other residents
Cultural ties	Illness/Dementia
Contracts/Leases	Building codes
Employment	Pets
Community ties	Identity
Too noisy/Fast	Too quiet/Slow
Wheelchair access	Disability

PLAN TWO
Don't move–improve.

Be prepared to assist aging family members who want to remain in their own homes. Ac-
commodating an aging relative's current and future lifestyle needs will lessen the caregiving
demands on you. In anticipation of any physical and psychological impairments, you can
adapt your elder's home environment to ensure safety and security while enhancing
his/her need for independence.

    Take a walking tour of the home accompanied by your relative. Write down observations and ideas on a notepad. Your common goal is to customize his/her living environment to meet current and future lifestyle needs. If your elder uses a wheelchair and/or motorized scooter, sit in the vehicle and take the tour from that perspective.

Plan to modify the home environment while creating a system of support so that aging family members can remain as self-sufficient as possible. For any major home construction, first consider the zoning laws and building codes.

Caregivers can expect to help their elders with . . .

Interior and exterior repairs
Home maintenance
Housekeeping
Heavy lifting
Shopping and errands
Transportation
Cooking
Personal care
Health care

Caregivers can expect to modify . . .

Bathrooms
Kitchen
Door widths, knobs, and locks
Lighting sources
Light switches
Shelf and counter heights
Appliance control panels and dials
Handles and window cranks
Telephone systems
Closet systems

Caregivers can expect to add . . .

First-floor bathroom and bedroom
Levers to replace knobs
Handrails and grab bars
Ramps
Lifting platforms

Caregivers can expect to buy . . .

Large-faced clocks, timers, thermostats
Glow-in-the-dark clocks
Talking clocks
Whistling tea kettles
Nonskid rugs, slippers, and socks
Handheld or clip-on fans
Adjustable furniture and bed
Night-lights
Illuminated light switches
Programmable thermostats
Verbal-command systems
Cordless telephones
Telephone voice mail service
Beepers
Emergency paging systems and call buttons
Room monitors
Medical alert bracelets or necklaces
Automatic turn-off appliances
Remote-control devices
"Reaching" devices
Microwave and toaster oven
Electric hand-mixers
Hearing aid
Shower and bath stool
Raised toilet seat
Home hospital equipment
Walkers and canes
Wheelchair
Flat rather than thick carpeting
Smoke/Carbon monoxide detectors
Nonbreakable glasses and dishes
Rubber-handled kitchen utensils
Bed tray
Luggage and grocery cart

Caregivers can expect to create support systems for . . .

Homemaker services
Personal care services
Home health care
Quality of life

PLAN THREE
**Learn which assisted and nonassisted living options best suit
your elder's housing needs now and in the future.**

Where an aging family member lives depends on many factors—health, money, safety, family and community support services, and preference. Here are some housing suggestions to serve as a guide in the decision-making process:

Shared housing is an arrangement when two or more related or unrelated people live together in the same house or apartment and share expenses. Tenants have private bedrooms, share the rest of the house, and may be able to arrange an exchange of services for rent.

ECHO housing (elder cottage housing opportunity) is the placement of a pre-built, independently run cottage on the private property of family or friends. Cottage units can be rented or purchased. Building codes and zoning laws regulate the possibility of this option.

Retirement communities (homes, condos, apartments, retirement hotels, mobile homes, cooperative housing) provide age-segregated, independent living units and offer personal care services, social activities, and limited nursing supervision. Retirement communities vary significantly in costs and benefits offered and are not subject to any particular regulation.

Assisted-living facilities (residential care facilities, rest homes, homes for the aged, board and care facilities) provide some personal care and nursing supervision, medication monitoring, social opportunities, meals, and housekeeping. These facilities appeal to elders who can no longer live at home, yet do not need professional nursing care. Residents are physically and mentally able to handle their daily needs. Sliding-scale placement is available in most states. Facilities are generally licensed by the state department of social services.

Life-care retirement communities (continuing care retirement communities) offer eligible individuals the option to buy or lease an apartment unit and are guaranteed care in a skilled nursing facility as part of the price of admission. When the leasing option is chosen, extended health-care services may vary. Entrance fees and monthly charges typically accompany this option. Waiting lists are usually long. Life-care facilities are state-licensed.

Group homes (congregate housing) are run by cities, profit and nonprofit groups such as religious organizations. This option usually requires that the resident is self-sufficient. Services provided include meals, housekeeping, transportation, social and recreational activities. Homes may or may not be regulated, depending on state laws. Financial assistance may be offered through the local public housing office.

Public housing is obtainable through the local housing authority. Homes and apartments are available throughout cities where landlords agree to accept prearranged, reduced rent. Waiting lists are long.

Adult foster care are single-family residences in which nonrelated elders live with a foster family that provides meals, housekeeping, and personal care.

Intermediate care facilities provide residence to elders finding it difficult to cope with activities of daily living and who need assistance managing medications. Elders in this setting may be in transition between hospital and home.

Skilled nursing facilities (nursing home, convalescent hospital) provide continuous skilled nursing care for those requiring twenty-four-hour medical attention. Caregivers can take advantage of this housing option if a short-term stay is all that is needed. Federal law prohibits nursing facilities to ask Medicare or Medicaid recipients for a deposit as a condition of admittance. Facilities are licensed by the state department of health services.

Elder housing options are listed in the yellow pages under Health Services, Homes— Residential Care, Hospitals, Nursing Homes, Rest Homes, and Retirement. Seek referrals from the hospital discharge planner or a geriatric social worker.

PLAN FOUR
Proceed with caution when considering a retirement facility.

If your aging family member is considering a retirement facility option, assist in asking specific questions and making astute observations:

- Location is important: Make sure the facility is close enough for friends and family to visit on a regular basis.
- Inquire about the possibility of waiting lists.
- Obtain all contracts, financial reports, resident rules and regulations and have them reviewed by an attorney or trusted advisor.
- Get proof of the facility's state license and accreditation certification.
- Ask to see a copy of the last inspection report.
- Visit all facilities under consideration.
- Visit several times, both during the day and at nighttime.
- Do a background check on who owns and manages the facility.
- Request copies of staff resumes. Arrange staff interviews.
- Use the services of an ombudsman (an advocate for retirement residents) to inquire about any past resident and family complaints and lawsuits.
- Obtain personal comments from at least three residents and their families.

During your visit use all your senses. Ask yourself . . .

Am I in a safe, comfortable, pleasant place?
Is the staff cheerful and friendly?
Are there odors I don't recognize or like?
Are the rooms well kept and nicely furnished? Homey?
Is the kitchen clean? Refrigerator clean and stocked?
Are dishes, pots, and pans clean?
Is the overall facility clean? Organized? Secure? Bug-free?
Are smoke and carbon monoxide detectors and fire extinguishers visible?
Does every room, including bathrooms, have an emergency call system?
Are bathrooms and showers properly maintained and stocked?
Are all rooms wheelchair accessible?
Are telephones within reach of wheelchair-bound residents?
Plenty of handrails and grab bars?
Are floors slippery?

Are heating and cooling systems working? Adequate?

Is there an out-of-doors area for residents to sit and walk?

Are the buildings and grounds well kept? Chipped paint? Lawn mowed? Snow shoveled? Sidewalks and curbs cracked or uneven?

Make sure things are in working order . . .

- Open doors, drawers, and windows.
- Turn on lights.
- Press emergency call buttons.
- Turn on televisions and radios.
- See if the telephones work.

Observe residents . . .

Are there bruises on the residents' arms and legs?

Are they neatly dressed? Wandering? Sitting aimlessly in halls?

Are they active? Happy?

Are they making use of the out-of-doors area?

Ask questions of the facility director . . .

On what grounds can I cancel housing contracts?

What is the staff-to-resident ratio?

Do volunteers work here? What is their turnover rate?

Have your staff and volunteers undergone specialized training?

How are workers and volunteers supervised?

What is the current occupancy rate?

Are residents required to carry health insurance?

Who monitors medications? What is the monitoring procedure?

Who evaluates resident illnesses?

How are medical emergencies handled?

Will the family doctor be able to continue to care for our family member?

How available are staff doctors and nurses?

How is the family kept informed? How often?

Do residents receive their own newsletter?

Can residents choose their own menus?

Are intergenerational activities available on a regular basis?

What specific social and exercise programs are provided?

Does the facility have family and resident support groups?

Is there a resident and family council that handles concerns?

How do you deal with problems between roommates?

What is the security system?

Are fire drills held regularly?

What are the smoking rules? Alcohol-use rules?

How long will the facility hold a room for a hospitalized resident?

Is transportation for residents provided?

Is there access to telephones for the residents?

Are postage stamps and incoming and outgoing mail services available?

Who is responsible for the resident's personal shopping?

Does each resident have an individual savings account for incidentals?

How are residents' religious needs met?

Does the facility offer educational classes?

Does the facility offer physical therapy?

Does the facility regularly celebrate holidays? Birthdays?

Are the bedrooms furnished?

May residents furnish their rooms with their own furniture?

Are linens provided?

How are personal laundry needs handled?

Is housekeeping provided?

Are assistants available to help the residents with getting dressed? Walking? Eating?

Can residents control their own heat/air-conditioning in their rooms?

Can residents have televisions in their rooms?

Is storage space available?

Does the facility offer personal care services such as hair styling?

Are pets allowed?

Ask specific financial questions . . .

What are the total monthly costs?

What is not included in the monthly costs? What is included?

What determines a rate increase? How often? When was the last one?

Do residents have any protection if fees go beyond their budget?

How are residents informed of rate increases?

What costs are covered by Medicare? Medicaid? Veteran's benefits?

What costs are covered by the resident's health insurance?
How are monthly payments made?
Are refunds available? Under what conditions?

Ask specific questions of the life-care retirement community . . .

Is the community accredited by a professional organization? Which one?
Are entrance fees refundable? Under what circumstances?
What are the resident's rights under remarriage? Must the new spouse meet requirements and pay an entrance fee?
What fees do residents continue to pay if they are sent to nursing units?
If one spouse is sent to the nursing unit, does the remaining spouse have to move to a smaller unit? Is there a change in the fee structure?
What is the plan to accommodate future high costs of nursing and health care services?
Does the facility have a cash reserve?
What are the future expansion and refurbishing building plans? How will this affect the residents' fees?
How are residents kept informed of the community's financial status?

Obtain complete, audited financial statements from the facility director. Have these statements reviewed by an attorney or trusted financial advisor. If the director refuses to comply or does not have a financial statement, seek housing elsewhere. Get *written* copies of all verbal and nonverbal agreements.

If any facility under consideration restricts visiting hours, it may have something to hide. Make astute observations for the existence of elder abuse—physical, verbal, medical, and emotional abuse and neglect, misuse of restraints both physically and chemically, and personal property abuse.

PLAN FIVE
Know what's in store before you ask your elder to move in with you.

Sometimes well-meaning family members insist that their aging relatives move in with them without full consideration of what can happen. The most serious stories include elder abuse and neglect, the fastest growing crime in America today. The arrangement of sharing one's home with an aging family member is likely to stir ambivalent feelings for everyone involved.

If you and your elder are thinking about combining households, discuss the following *before* the move:

Ask your elder . . .

Do you want to move in?
Do you want to share a household with these family members?
How long are you prepared to live here?
Are there any relationship conflicts that need to be resolved before you move in?
Are you prepared to help with any costs?

Ask family residents . . .

Does anyone resent this living arrangement?
How do you feel about this relative?
How do you feel about spending time with this relative on a daily basis?
What adjustments would you have to make to your lifestyle?
Is it possible for you to treat the elder as a full member of the family, not to be ignored or isolated?

Ask yourself . . .

Is this decision based on guilt or a sense of obligation?
How will this decision affect my lifestyle, my relationships, my job, my activities inside and outside of my home?
How would I feel about spending time with my relative on a daily basis?
Is there a plan in place if I am unavailable to care for my elder?
Are there ways for my elder to contribute to the family and feel needed?
Is there a plan to preserve privacy and autonomy for everyone?
What is the plan when mood swings set in?
Is my family financially and emotionally stable?
Is there any other member of the family who currently requires a lot of attention and time?
Are these plans realistic?

Discuss with the family members . . .

The plan for family status changes—loss of income, divorce, death, marriages, births, pets, vacations.
Family and friends' visitation rights.

Elder's access to a full range of activities—inside and outside of the home—
   places of worship, friends, relatives, shopping, entertainment.
Sharing responsibilities.
What are the costs and who pays?

PLAN SIX
Consider the shared housing option.

Sharing a home with people outside of the immediate family is fast becoming a practical
living arrangement, replacing the idea of living strictly with relatives.

Doubling-up means cutting housing costs, sharing chores, and providing an opportunity of friendship, support, and love. This form of sharing has its problems; living close
to others always does. To live alone creates isolation. As your elder ages, the ability to get
along with others will become increasingly important.

There are plenty of people available to share a home: another elderly person, grandchildren, college students, nursing students, foreign exchange students, single parents
with kids, friends, neighbors, co-workers, and church members.

PLAN SEVEN
Plan for a smooth transition when it comes to moving your elder.

Eight weeks before . . .

• Shop for a moving company.
• Get three estimates and compare services.
• Ask about price breaks and low-season discounts.
• Ask how payments are made.
• Ask about insurance for damaged goods.

One month before . . .

• Request moving checklist from moving company.
• Review the moving agreement details.
• Start packing. Discard, distribute, and donate unwanted possessions.
• Photograph valuable possessions before having them moved.

• Fill out change of address cards. (Get forms from the post office.)
• Transfer prescriptions to the new pharmacy.
• Arrange disconnection and connection of utilities and telephone.
• Arrange the transportation of pets and plants.
• Reserve the elevator in high-rise buildings.

Final week . . .

• Make arrangements for payment of movers.
• Arrange for packers to start boxing items to be moved.

Moving day . . .

• Be home when movers arrive.
• Watch as belongings are inventoried, packed, and loaded on truck.
• Check the bill of lading.
• Review destination with movers.
• Give movers telephone number, backup telephone number, and where you can
  be reached on other end.

Delivery day . . .

• Be home when movers arrive.
• Be prepared to pay with cash/money order upon delivery.
• Keep moving-related receipts for tax purposes.

Low Cost/Free Resources

Universities with gerontology centers may have the names of people and facilities who can provide information about housing options, home safety, and chore services.

The **area agency on aging** can provide information on federal, state, city, and county programs aimed at setting up support systems for those who want to stay where they are and live independently.

Hospital discharge planners and the **long-term care ombudsman** (who can be located through your local area agency on aging) can assist family with decisions about appropriate levels of care and housing.

For an evaluation of how your elder's home can be adapted to safer, easier living, contact the **Visiting Nurses Association.**

To locate **advocacy organizations** regarding nursing home residents and their families, consult the local chapters of United Way, The United Hospital Fund, AARP, Gray Panthers, and long-term care ombudsman.

The **U.S. Department of Housing and Urban Development (HUD)** is the government agency which provides low-cost housing. Contact the housing authority of your city or investigate on website *http://hud/gov/senior.html.*

ORGANIZATIONS

Access Living
310 S. Peoria St., Suite 201, Chicago, IL 60607, (312) 226-5900

American Association of Homes and Services for the Aging
901 E St., NW, Suite 500, Washington, DC 20004, (202) 783-2242, (800) 508-9442
Website *http://www.spry.org/aahsa.htm*

American Rehab
1910 Association Dr., Suite 200, Reston, VA 22091, (703) 648-9300

Assisted Living Facility Association of America
9401 Lee Highway, Suite 402, Fairfax, VA 22031, (703) 691-8100

Concerned Relatives of Nursing Home Patients
3130 Mayfield Road, Suite 209 W, Cleveland Heights, OH 44118, (216) 321-0403

National Association for Home Care
519 C St., NE, Washington, DC 20002, (202) 547-7424
Website *http://www.nahc.org/*

National Center for State Long-Term Care Ombudsman Resources
1225 I St., NW, Suite 725, Washington, DC 20005, (202) 898-2578

National Citizens Coalition for Nursing Home Reform
1424 16th St., NW, Suite 202, Washington, DC 20002, (202) 332-2275

National Council of Senior Citizens
1331 F St., NW, Suite 800, Washington, DC 20004, (202) 347-8800

National Council on Aging
409 Third St., SW, Washington, DC 20024, (202) 479-1200

National Eldercare Institute on Housing and Supportive Services
University of Southern California Andrus Gerontology Center,
Los Angeles, CA 90089, (310) 740-1364

National Foundation for Retirement Living
184 Gloucester St., Annapolis, MD 21403, (800) 626-6767

National Shared Housing Resource Center
321 E. 25th St., Baltimore, MD 21218, (410) 235-4454

Action Checklist

HOME SUITE HOME	To Do By	Completed
Consider possible change in housing (Plan One).	_____	❑
Set housing goals . . .		
short-term	_____	❑
long-term	_____	❑
Determine home modifications (Plan Two) . . .		
short-term	_____	❑
long-term	_____	❑
Check laws and codes for home remodeling.	_____	❑
Determine caregiver support systems . . .		
homemaker	_____	❑
personal care	_____	❑
home health care	_____	❑
quality of life	_____	❑
Review housing options (Plan Three) . . .		
Family member's home	_____	❑
ECHO housing	_____	❑
Retirement residence	_____	❑
Life-Care/Retirement	_____	❑
Housing	_____	❑
Group home	_____	❑
Public housing	_____	❑
Intermediate care	_____	❑
Skilled nursing facility	_____	❑
Shared housing (Plan Six)	_____	❑
Create facility questions and checklists (Plan Four).	_____	❑
Take family consensus before asking elder to move in (Plan Five).	_____	❑
Develop moving strategy (Plan Seven).	_____	❑

Chapter 8

SAFE AND SECURE

Minimize Distress over Distance

A growing number of family caregivers assist aging relatives from long distances, creating a disturbing mixture of anxiety and fear. More than half of the adult children of aging parents live at least 100 miles away. The rise in long-distance family caregiving is a consequence of a society on the move. Family members frequently relocate to pursue professional and personal interests and opportunities as a way to improve the quality of their lives.

At the same time, family caregivers are increasingly concerned that they won't be able to respond immediately to an eldercare emergency and their aging relatives are afraid of the consequences. How, then, do we help our elders to balance their desire to remain at home—measurably independent—while assuring for their safety and security?

The answer requires family members to reach a consensus on making the home a safe place, learning how to recognize and avoid popular money scams, and creating informal and formal systems of support. The action plans listed in this portion of the planner will specifically guide you in ensuring for your elder's safety.

However, no matter how much you plan for your elder's safety, the feelings of anxiety may remain. When these feelings surface, sometimes just picking up the telephone and calling your relative to hear his or her familiar voice may be all the reassurance you need.

MINIMIZE DISTRESS OVER DISTANCE

- A major fear of the elderly is being helpless if something happened at home and no one would know.
- According to the House Select Committee on Aging, elder abuse is up a dramatic 50 percent. The most likely victims are women over seventy-five years of age.
- Scam artists play on aging people's fears about maintaining a comfortable lifestyle on a fixed income. The telephone is the most popular vehicle of choice for committing fraud.

Help your aging family members avoid becoming a crime and accident statistic with basic prevention strategies.

Objectives

After completing Minimize Distress over Distance you will be able to:

Recognize existing or potential hazards in your relative's home.

Initiate safety and security precautions.

Create check-in systems.

Detect signs of elder abuse and neglect.

Identify potential and existing scams, frauds, and con-artists.

PLAN ONE
Home safety is no accident.

Creating a safe and mobile living space for our aging family members will help them maintain their independence. Be aware, however, that too much cleaning up can confuse a person who relies on a series of routines and memory.

Following are things you can check on to make your relative's home as safe and secure as possible:

Throughout the home . . .

- Electric cords are in good working condition and safely tucked away.
- Extension cords are not overloaded.
- Smoke and carbon monoxide detectors are present and working.
- Electrical outlets are not warm to the touch.
- Home is well lit—inside and out.
- Night lights are present in hallways, stairwells, bedrooms, bathrooms.
- Electric heaters are placed away from curtains, rugs, furnishings.
- Electric appliances are a safe distance from water.
- Fireplace chimneys are clear of accumulation and checked yearly.
- Light switches are present at the top and bottom of stairs.
- Stairwells are well lit.
- Light switches are located near room entrances.
- Stairways are free of objects.
- Stair handrails are present and sturdy.
- Stairs are marked for visibility with contrasting tape.
- Steps are even and uniform in size and height.
- Floors are not slippery or highly polished.
- Carpeting, linoleum, plastic stair treads are secure.
- Carpets are free of holes and snags.
- Carpet edges are securely fastened.
- Water temperature is reduced to prevent scalding.
- Water faucets are clearly marked hot and cold.
- House smoking rules are established.
- Rope ladders are available on upper levels.
- Furnace is checked yearly.
- Room furniture patterns give easy access to doors and windows.

- Rooms are free of floor clutter.
- Stairs and pathways are free of objects.
- Drawers, doors, and windows open and shut easily.
- Flashlights are available in every room.
- Glow tape is adhered on items to identify them in the dark.
- Cleaners and poisons are clearly marked.
- Step stools are sturdy.
- Window and door locks are secure and operating.
- Medications are properly stored and usage instructions are written down.
- First-aid kit is available and contains up-to-date supplies.

In the kitchen . . .

- Dishes and food are stored on lower shelves.
- Towels and curtains are away from the stove.
- Lighting is sufficient over stove, sink, and countertops.
- Radio and electric appliances are a distance from the sink.
- "Off" indicators on stove and appliances are clearly marked with brightly colored tape.
- A telephone is in the kitchen.
- Emergency telephone numbers are displayed near telephone and on the refrigerator.
- Fire extinguisher is in easy reach and in working order.
- Whistling tea kettle and food-timers are in use.
- Food is properly stored in freezer.
- Food is used before the expiration date.
- Plastic, easy-open containers and dishes replace glassware.
- Heavy pots or pans are replaced with lighter ones.
- Handles on pots and pans are sturdy.
- Pot-holder mitts are available and used.
- Refrigerator and stove are in good working order.
- Sturdy step stool is available.
- Pet dishes are tucked away from walking path.

In the bedroom . . .

- Lamps and light switches are within reach of bed.
- Electric blanket is in good working order.

• Telephone is accessible next to bed.
• Emergency telephone list is near the telephone.
• Flashlight and whistle are near bed.
• Medications are away from the nightstand.
• Bed is the appropriate height.

In the bathroom . . .

• Nonskid decals and rubber mats are in tub and shower.
• Floor rugs are secure.
• Grab bars and handrails are next to toilet and in tub and shower.
• Handrails are secure.
• Shower and tub stools are present.
• There is telephone access in bathroom.

Home exterior . . .

• Tools and yard equipment are safely and securely stored.
• Solvents, paints, sprays are clearly marked.
• Goggles are worn when using power equipment.
• Stair rails are secure.
• There are clear, safe walking paths and no holes in concrete.
• Leaves and snow are cleared away.
• There is telephone access while outside.
• Stairs are replaced with ramps if necessary.
• Porch lights are in working order.

PLAN TWO
Help aging family members play it safe.

The following safety precautions save lives.
    Basic safety tips . . .

• Dry hands and feet when using tools and appliances.
• Wear short sleeves when cooking.
• Plan two ways to get out of the house during an emergency.
• Know how to change fuses and circuit breakers.

- Keep a spare set of house keys, car keys, and eyeglasses.
- Read directions before installing and operating appliances and equipment.
- Display emergency phone numbers near telephones and on refrigerator.
- Display list of medications near telephone and on refrigerator.
- Take drugs responsibly.
- Purchase long-handled grippers, sponges, dusters for easy reach.
- Use a cordless telephone for easy access.
- Wear nonskid slippers, socks, and low-heeled shoes.
- Beware of robes and pajamas that are too long.
- Never store items on stairs.
- Get assistance when changing light bulbs.

Guarding against burglary and other potential harm . . .

- Never keep large amounts of cash in the house.
- Telephone answer machine message should not indicate that no one is home or on vacation.
- Be discrete about letting others know you live alone.
- Do not open the door automatically.
- Never let strangers use the telephone.
- Do not let service people in house if you did not initiate the service.
- Ask for proper identification from delivery and service people.
- Install peepholes and deadbolts.
- Befriend helpful, watchful neighbors.
- Participate in family, neighbor, and volunteer check-in systems.
- Draw blinds and drapes at night.
- Lock windows, doors, garages, gates, and car doors.
- Do not leave notes on door when going out.
- Leave lights, radio, or TV on when going out.
- Do not put keys in the mailbox or under doormat.
- Report all crimes and suspicious activities.
- Travel in pairs.
- Carry homeowner or renter insurance.
- Engrave valuables with Social Security number.
- Keep written inventory, videos, or photographs of possessions.
- Keep original documents and photocopies separate.
- Store important documents in a safe place.

• Store valuables in a safe or bank safe-deposit box.
• Inquire about the bank's policy on insuring safe-deposit box.

When going away on an extended trip . . .

• Use light timing devices inside and outside the home.
• Notify neighbors and police of your absence.
• Suspend newspapers, have post office hold mail.
• Arrange for lawn to be mowed, snow shoveled.
• Leave radio or television on.
• Make sure major appliances are off except refrigerator.
• Lock and secure all doors and windows.
• Store ladders inside.
• Disconnect the automatic garage door opener.
• Put valuables in locked storage.
• Leave phone numbers of where you can be reached with family and friends.

While walking outdoors . . .

• Walk purposefully, confidently, and keep alert to surroundings.
• Wear shoes that promote balance and easy walking.
• Don't overload yourself with packages.
• Resist wearing a shoulder-purse.
• Do not drape purse strap across torso. Carry purse like a football, close to the body.
• Walk in well-lit areas.
• Have keys in hand when approaching doors and car.
• Put a wide rubber band around wallets and purses.
• Do not walk, jog, or bike with headphones.
• Carry a whistle or a loud alarm.
• If in danger, yell "Fire!" or "Police!"
• Get license plate number of all suspicious cars and file a report.
• Avoid public transportation in very early or late hours.

While driving . . .

• Check front, back seat, and rear of car before entering.
• Keep doors locked, windows up.
• Stow purse on floor behind driver's seat. Put all packages in the trunk.

- Keep a disposable camera in glove compartment to document damage.
- If being followed, drive to police station, fire station, or hospital emergency room entrance. Honk car horn to summon help.
- Keep car in gear at stop signs and traffic lights.
- Travel well-lit streets.
- Keep emergency items in trunk—hat, gloves, long-underwear, shovel, rags, water, throw rug, battery charger, spare tire, flashlight, umbrella, maps.
- Never pick up hitchhikers.
- If car breaks down, move car off to side, raise hood, turn on flashers, get back in car, and wait for help.

Safe banking and shopping . . .

- Have monthly checks deposited directly into account.
- Do not display large sums of cash.
- Avoid carrying cash.
- Don't get cash from outdoor mechanical bank-teller systems.
- Never leave purse unattended.

For safety devices and services see the yellow pages under . . .

Paging and signaling equipment	Burglar alarm systems
Radio communication equipment	Security
Safety equipment	Locks and locksmiths
Fire extinguishers	Fire protection/Alarm systems
Smoke detection equipment	Protection devices
Flame proofing	Medical alarms

PLAN THREE
Create check-in systems.

Any safety check should include an assessment of your elder's mental health. Depression and anxiety, for instance, often increase the risk of accidents.

Whether your aging relative lives independently at home, in a group or nursing home setting, create ongoing check-in systems with family members, neighbors, community members, church groups, schools, volunteers, and professional care providers. Be sure all designated persons have keys to your relative's home.

If your relative becomes defensive about the amount of attention he/she is receiving, offer the following reasons for your actions . . .

- To ensure safety and security
- To detect elder abuse and neglect
- To uncover hidden problems
- To avoid a crisis
- To protect his/her rights
- To offer peace of mind knowing someone is there

Check-in systems include . . .

Telephone reassurance programs. A telephone network that calls each day to check on a person's well-being. Failure to answer brings a second call within minutes. No answer results in a call to a designated person who goes to the individual's home.

Phone Alert League (PAL). A community program offering service to anyone living alone. If the person does not call PAL between a certain time, PAL will call and send someone to the person's residence.

Carrier Alert. Elderly people can register to participate in this program with post office. A sticker is placed inside the mailbox to alert postman in the event of accumulating mail. The post office then calls the phone number on the sticker or the emergency number listed at the post office.

Emergency response device. Permits an individual to call for assistance. A variety of products are on the market. Get references from the hospital discharge planner.

In-person check-in. Ask a neighbor or friend to check in on your aging relative on a regular basis. Pay them for their time. If they don't accept money, buy them small gifts to show your appreciation.

Vial of Life program. Available through the county sheriff's office. Vital emergency data regarding an individual's health care is stored in a vial in the refrigerator. A sticker on the door alerts emergency personnel that the information is there.

Friendly visitors programs. Provide regular visitors to homes and nursing home facilities. Universities and church groups often participate.

Senior escort programs. The elderly receive transportation and companionship to community programs and doctor appointments. Contact the area agency on aging and family service organizations.

Ombudsman. Resolves complaints and investigates allegations of patient abuse. Listed in the telephone book white pages under long-term care ombudsman or through your local area agency on aging.

Plan Four
Get the facts about elder abuse and neglect.

The aging of our society as a whole presents many challenges. A substantial number of elderly people are cared for by adult children, spouses, friends, and volunteers. Elder abuse and neglect is not a new problem and can be found anywhere—in the home, residential facilities, and hospitals. Abusers include family members, professional caregivers, volunteers, employees, and strangers.

Abuse and neglect may be due to the caregiver's lack of knowledge or capacity to care for the aging person. Abuse and neglect also can be a symptom of a stressed family or a long-standing difficult parent/child relationship.

Unintentional failure to fulfill a caregiving obligation, name-calling, ignoring, threatening, isolating, exploiting of funds, physical abuse, denial of food and water, medication mismanagement, failure to provide health care, violation of rights (such as opening mail), denial of freedom of speech or the freedom to worship are all forms of abuse and neglect.

Caregivers should be on the constant lookout for signs of elder abuse and neglect and report their concerns immediately.

Plan Five
Outsmart the con-artists.

An elderly person may become vulnerable to manipulation by family, nonfamily, and strangers out of loneliness, fear, greed, and a willingness to believe what they are told.

Danger signs include . . .

- Door-to-door salespeople
- Unexpected visits from people with official-sounding titles
- Unsolicited phone calls from people asking questions about money, family, burglar alarms, credit cards, checking accounts
- Unsolicited money offers and money transfers from people who identify themselves as friends of the family, bank officials, insurance agents, law officers, and city inspectors
- Unsolicited offers for home repairs and "free home tests"
- "Opportunities of a lifetime" offers
- Urgent, official-looking government documents that come in the mail
- Offers promising 20 percent to 100 percent return on investments within a short period of time and return is guaranteed
- "Act now" sales pitches and any sales with a sense of urgency
- Person selling winning lottery tickets
- Investments located in faraway places—Alaskan oil, for example
- Post-It notes attached to newspaper articles arriving in unmarked envelopes—making it look as though someone you know is recommending the product or service
- Mobile health labs offering elderly "free" health-screening services not covered by Medicare
- Mailings or salespeople using scare tactics
- Ads showing fistfuls of dollars and money trees
- Crooks who buy uniform jackets worn by police officers and security guards
- Early morning (1 a.m. to 4 a.m.) phone calls

Avoid being taken . . .

- Never open door to strangers. Not even so-called city inspectors, telephone repair workers, or utility company employees if you did not initiate the visit. Call the police.
- Give a post office official all suspicious-looking mail so they can track down offenders.
- Show family members all official-looking mail.
- Never give credit card or bank account numbers over the phone.
- Keep Social Security numbers confidential.
- Be fully aware of the costs involved with 900 telephone numbers. Read the fine print.

- Beware of bogus products sold through 900 phone numbers.
- Have family members meet all new "friends."
- Never authorize services without up-front, signed estimates.
- Have a trusted advisor review all estimates before authorizing work.
- Never give strangers money for any reason.
- Don't discuss personal finances with strangers.
- Know that con-artists create an aura of legitimacy by paying "satisfied customers" to lie about the company.
- Check with trusted family members or financial advisor before making any investments.
- Never spend money to claim a prize.
- Buy art, antiques, jewelry, and collections from reputable dealers who provide insurance to cover the purchase price of the item if value is misrepresented. Ask other collectors and museum curators for referrals.
- Don't buy goods offered out of the backs of trucks and autos. You might be buying stolen property.
- Don't pay or accept unsolicited C.O.D. packages.
- Check references and credentials of all service providers.
- Avoid deals you don't understand.
- Never take advice from someone who is trying to sell you something.
- Hang up immediately on all unsolicited sales calls and calls from strangers.
- Don't be embarrassed to report frauds.
- Ask your physician about the reputation of any "free" mobile health labs in question.
- Do not endorse "gift" checks, coupons, sweepstakes entries, or rebates sent by mail from unknown sources. You may be signing an agreement or appointing some unknown person or company to provide unwanted services.
- Check all warranties—length of time covered, what coverage includes and excludes, the replacement parts policy—on any major purchase, new or used.
- Find out if service provider individuals and companies are bonded and licensed. Avoid wandering "fix-it" types.
- Never donate cash to a charity. Write a check and get a receipt.
- Call the Better Business Bureau, chamber of commerce, state office on consumer affairs, state's attorney's office, or state's security office on reliability of business and charities. Ask about license requirements and disciplinary records.

Don't fall for popular scams . . .

• Alzheimer's cures
• Medicare home medical equipment telephone sales
• Arthritis remedies
• Instant weight-loss schemes
• Sexual stimulants
• Baldness remedies
• Nutritional cure-alls
• Wrinkle removers
• Unsolicited home repair
• Home tests like radon schemes
• Lottery and sweepstakes swindles
• Funeral home investments
• Mail-order life insurance policies

If money has changed hands, call the . . .

• Company and demand return of money
• Police
• U.S. attorney's office
• Federal Trade Commission
• Better Business Bureau
• Chamber of commerce
• State securities office
• District attorney's office

Low Cost/Free Resources

Telecommunication Device for the Deaf (TDD) and **Braille TDDs** are available for telephone customers with hearing and sight disabilities. Contact the Special Needs Center of the telephone company.

To participate in a **self-defense class,** find listings in the telephone yellow pages under Martial Arts Instruction or call the area agency on aging to find classes especially for seniors.

A free **home safety guide** is available at a nearby AAA Motor Club office.

If you suspect elder abuse and neglect, call the department of social services' **adult protection services.** Contact the **state long-term care ombudsman** for abuse and neglect in residential and nursing home care facilities. In an emergency call 911.

Have the **gas** and **electric company** do a home survey on appliances and make energy-saving suggestions. Most major utility companies have a toll-free action line for questions. Get the telephone number for your particular state from the utility company.

The **police** or **sheriff's department** will pay a home visit to show how security can be improved.

Ask a **fire official** to visit the home to check on fire hazards. Let official know if your relative smokes and what can be done about it.

For an evaluation of how your elder's home can be adapted for safer, easier living, contact the **Visiting Nurses Association.**

Some communities have **neighborhood watch** programs. Call the police department to find out more.

To learn **CPR** (cardiopulmonary resuscitation) contact the American Heart Association, American Red Cross, or the fire station for location of courses. Check the yellow pages under First-aid Instruction.

If you have questions about air quality, or solid or hazardous waste, contact the **state department of environmental protection.**

ORGANIZATIONS

Council of Better Business Bureaus, Inc.
4200 Wilson Blvd., Suite 800, Arlington, VA 22203, (703) 276-0100
Website *http://www.bbb.org/bbb*

National Safety Council
1121 Spring Lake Dr., Itasca, IL 60143, (800) 621-7619

National Fraud Information Center
PO Box 65868, Washington, DC 20035-5868, (800) 876-7060
Website *http://www.fraud.org*

Action Checklist

MINIMIZE DISTRESS OVER DISTANCE	To Do By	Completed
Set safe and secure goals . . .		
short-term	_____	❑
long-term	_____	❑
Review home hazards (Plan One) . . .		
throughout home	_____	❑
kitchen	_____	❑
bedroom	_____	❑
bathroom	_____	❑
exterior	_____	❑
garage	_____	❑
Have elder's home surveyed by . . .		
police	_____	❑
fire official	_____	❑
electric company	_____	❑
gas company	_____	❑
Implement safety precautions (Plan Two) . . .		
at home	_____	❑
on an extended trip	_____	❑
walking	_____	❑
driving	_____	❑
banking	_____	❑
shopping	_____	❑
Create check-in systems (Plan Three) . . .		
telephone	_____	❑
carrier alert	_____	❑
beepers	_____	❑
visitors	_____	❑
lifeline	_____	❑
vial of life	_____	❑

MINIMIZE DISTRESS OVER DISTANCE	To Do By	Completed
escorts	_____	❑
ombudsman	_____	❑
Check for abuse and neglect (Plan Four).	_____	❑
Plan to ward off con-artists (Plan Five).	_____	❑
Elders with hearing/sight disabilities have access to a telephone.	_____	❑
Know the telephone numbers of . . .		
police	_____	❑
fire	_____	❑
electric company	_____	❑
water company	_____	❑
gas company	_____	❑
plumber	_____	❑
electrician	_____	❑

Chapter 9

TRANSPORTATION

Steer Clear

Losing driving privileges in today's mobile society is a serious loss—emotionally and psychologically. When you take a license away, it typically results in fewer social contacts and an increasing dependence on others.

It's true we have to get high-risk elderly drivers off the road; but before you bring up the subject with aging family members, be sure your concern about their driving ability is well-founded. Ability, not age, is the determining factor.

To have the coordination to stop suddenly; to be able to see clearly night and day; to distinguish between light and dark areas, such as silhouettes of people crossing streets at dusk; to be mentally alert; to move arms, legs, and head easily; to be able to hear; to manage the use of drugs and alcohol; and to maintain the car to safety and licensing standards should be the basis of such conversations.

This section of the planner offers specific suggestions on getting impaired elderly drivers off the road. At the same time, paying attention to your communication approach is an essential part of the process. First, when dealing with sensitive topics (like driving), ask questions instead of making demands—*Do you ever get scared when you drive? Do you think you can see all right? Do other drivers make you nervous? Would you consider not driving at night anymore? Is your car expensive to maintain? Isn't parking getting more difficult and expensive these days?* This line of questioning will get them thinking about the subject. Second, decide what's best for you. If you feel that you and your family are not safe when riding as passengers in your elder's car, you have the right to decline his/her offer to drive. Third, offer to drive or have someone else take your relative where he/she wants to go.

Studies reveal that most elderly drivers quit when they are ready. Your goal is to gently remind them that you are concerned for their safety in these particularly dangerous times. This may be all that is necessary to help them make the decision to stop driving.

STEER CLEAR

- Countless drivers insist on getting behind the wheel while medicated.
- By age eighty-five and older, drivers have more serious-injury and fatal accidents per mile driven than teen drivers.
- Even if a person has 20/20 daytime vision, nighttime vision will have weakened considerably by the age of forty.
- Resistance, viewed positively, may mean an elderly driver continues to be self-reliant and is showing others that he/she is still in charge.

If someone you love is a hazardous driver, be prepared to take certain steps to eliminate a potentially serious danger.

Objectives

After completing Steer Clear you will be able to:

Prepare yourself for arguments and resistance.

Encourage elderly drivers to monitor their own ability to drive.

Suggest transportation options.

Minimize the potential for your elder to become isolated and inactive.

PLAN ONE
Use negotiating skills to get an impaired elderly driver off the road.

Currently there are no national standards to identify older drivers who have critical impairments. Ideally, your elderly family member will decide for himself/herself not to drive. Frustrated relatives, in the meantime, may resort to underhanded tactics like hiding the car keys and disabling the car. These drastic measures sacrifice trust, honesty, and maturity in your relationship with your elder.

If your relative has a bad driving record and he/she refuses to stop driving, first get the support of the whole family and arrange for professional backup. The doctor may be willing to discuss medical issues. NOTE: Don't expect much help from your elder's friends. They may be struggling with the same issue.

Be prepared for resistance and stubbornness. Instead of making demands, negotiate impaired elderly drivers off the road with these suggestions:

Ask your elder to agree to . . .

- Take the 55 Alive program offered by AARP. This course may even qualify a driver for an auto insurance discount.
- Consult radio highway reports before getting behind the wheel.
- Not drive while medicated or using alcohol.
- Not drive at night.
- Not drive in bad weather.
- Drive shorter distances.
- Avoid rush hours.
- Drive with the radio off, window slightly open to hear horns and sirens.
- Listen if anyone refuses or hesitates to drive with him/her.
- Stop driving if other drivers make him/her jumpy or nervous.
- Take public transportation, taxis, or let others drive.
- Take a professional driving assessment test provided by driving schools and the state department of motor vehicles office.
- Get regular eye and physical exams.
- Join an automobile club that offers road services.
- Buy raised car seats and seat pads if needed.
- Consider the high costs of maintaining the parking, payments, insurance, upkeep, licenses, fees, stickers, and gasoline.
- Acknowledge other potential dangers such as car jackers, drunk drivers, and speeders.

PLAN TWO
If all else fails, bring in the law.

If you have clear evidence that your relative is a danger to himself/herself and other drivers, there are legal steps you can take to alert authorities:

- Report impaired drivers to the department of motor vehicles. You may have to make a court appearance or you may be able to tell your concerns over the phone. Find out whether you can maintain your confidentiality and what consequences you face should you file a report.

- Ask the department of motor vehicles to send your elder notice to retake the driving exam. They will need this request in writing along with his/her name, address, date of birth, driver's license number, and vehicle license plate number.

- If your elder insists on driving while heavily medicated, ask the prescribing physician to send a letter of request to the department of motor vehicles to put a stop to his/her driving—temporarily or permanently. The doctor also may recommend that your elder discontinue driving because of physical and mental limitations.

PLAN THREE
Lessen the need to drive.

Door-to-door service is only a phone call away. Make these suggestions to eliminate unnecessary trips in the car:

- Call the customer service department of stores and ask for home assistance.
- Arrange for home delivery.
- Use reputable mail-order catalogues and have gifts wrapped and sent directly to recipient.
- Use direct deposit, automated bill paying, and money transfer banking services.
- Shop at home with TV and radio buying programs.
- Inquire about home visits from health-care and personal-care service providers, government services, and clergy.

PLAN FOUR
Supply your elder with transportation alternatives.

Following are suggestions on other ways to get around town:

Locate drivers and private transportation providers—family, friends, neighbors, church members, volunteers, students, and youth groups. Professional drivers can also be hired if finances allow.

Ask about transportation services supplied by health-care organizations, shopping malls, community transfer services, and government agencies.

Create a taxi fund. Encourage family members to contribute. Take advantage of senior citizen taxi discount coupons available in many communities.

Carpool to regularly scheduled activities and shopping excursions.

Supply your relative with public transportation maps and schedules. Senior citizen discounts are usually available.

Obtain handicapped transportation information by contacting specialized transport companies with door-to-door services.

PLAN FIVE
Prevent isolation.

Try as best you can to keep your aging family member connected with others:

- Invite your elder to regularly scheduled activities such as birthday parties, weekend entertainment, meals, and holiday celebrations.
- Arrange to have regular home visitors such as other family members, friends, children, pets, clergy, and volunteers.
- Suggest that your relative get involved in clubs and activities where participants carpool.

Low Cost/Free Resources

Contact the local **AAA Motor Club** and request information on older drivers, driving assessment programs, and traffic safety.

Contact the **American Red Cross** and ask about the volunteer drivers program that provides rides to and from medical appointments.

Specialized medical centers usually provide transportation to and from treatments. Call the **area agency on aging** or the **hospital discharge planner** director for details.

Some **shopping malls** provide transit services. Call them directly.

Many **senior centers** throughout the country provide transportation to social activities. Call the individual centers for more information.

Senior citizen taxi coupons are available in most communities. Call the area agency on aging.

ORGANIZATIONS

American Automobile Association
1000 AAA Dr., Heathrow, FL 32746, (407) 444-4300

American Automobile Association Foundation for Traffic Safety
12600 Fair Lakes Circle, Fairfax, VA 22033, (703) AAA-6000

Association of Driver Educators for the Disabled
(608) 884-8833

Auto Safety Hotline
(800) 424-9393

Community Transportation Association of America
Website *http://www.ctaa.org*

National Community Transportation Association of America
1440 New York Ave., NW, Suite 440, Washington, DC 20005, (202) 628-1480

Action Checklist

STEER CLEAR	To Do By	Completed
Set transportation goals . . .		
short-term	_____	❏
long-term	_____	❏
Monitor elder's ability to drive.	_____	❏
Discuss . . .		
driving course (Plan One)	_____	❏
driving conditions (Plan One)	_____	❏
alternatives (Plan Four)	_____	❏
Lessen the need to drive (Plan Three).	_____	❏
Create ways to be socially active (Plan Five).	_____	❏
Take legal action (Plan Two).	_____	❏
Know phone numbers of . . .		
auto insurance	_____	❏
auto club	_____	❏
motor vehicle department	_____	❏
Keep copy of elder's . . .		
auto insurance card	_____	❏
auto club card	_____	❏

Chapter 10

HEALTH AND WELLNESS

Taking Charge: Healthy Living Tips

Many of us know that proper diet and exercise help us take charge of our physical and mental well-being. We even are encouraged to ask questions of our health-care professionals if we don't fully understand their recommendations. Today's elderly, on the other hand, live by another set of health-care rules and roles. For the most part they were taught not to question their doctor's authority and may consequently believe that their health is solely in someone else's hands.

The practice of self-health care on the part of our aging family members most likely requires them to learn an entirely new set of behaviors. A lifetime of deep-rooted habits is difficult to change and the idea of taking charge of one's own health may not come easily. Instead of preaching the benefits of self-health care, a more effective approach uses family caregivers as a source of influence and information. We can demonstrate the process of eating right, we can explain how exercise has made a difference in our lives, we can tell them the joys of staying socially active.

Try to remember, however, that your elders will grasp this concept of self-health care only if they want to. Plenty of health-care information is available to them, but it is solely their decision to act upon it. At the least, you can use this section of the planner to help your elders make informed decisions about their health-care providers and their own health care. An educated consumer makes a big difference in health management and treatment options.

TAKING CHARGE: HEALTHY LIVING TIPS

- "Older means weaker" is a myth. Many types of strength remain constant throughout life. In general, muscle strength begins to decline only after age seventy.
- Thousands of deaths could be prevented if family members would learn which diseases run in their families.
- Half of all women experience urinary incontinence at some point in their lives, yet wait an average of nine years before getting help.
- Health is a means, not an end. Patients must assume a greater responsibility for their own health.

Paying the high cost of improper self-health care, financially and emotionally, is one of the most complex, difficult problems in this country. It *is* preventable.

Objectives

After completing Taking Charge: Healthy Living Tips you will be able to:

Encourage aging relatives to live a more healthy lifestyle.

Acquaint yourself with health-care professionals and the services they provide.

Combat your elder's inattention or overattention to his/her health.

PLAN ONE
Encourage your elder to live healthy and stay strong.

Aging is inevitable, disease and disability are not. Many health problems are preventable. The suggestions below are meant to serve as springboards for self-health care conversations with your elder.

Exercise. It is never too late to start. One-half hour of brisk walking four times a week has been shown to increase health substantially. More vigorous exercise improves mood states and self-esteem. Physical frailty can be reversed by exercise. To stay active, feet must be comfortable. Corns, bunions, and calluses are problems a good podiatrist can help remedy. Good shoes with proper support are essential.

Activities include . . .

Golf	Bike	Shuffleboard	Croquet
Swim	Bowl	Billiards	Weights
Jog	Garden	Racquetball	Aerobics
Walk	Dance	Softball	Aqua aerobics
Hike	Tennis	Lawn bowling	Yoga
Climb stairs	Badminton	Horseshoes	Stretch classes

Eat right. Read labels. Ask your doctor about a healthy weight for you. Women who gain just twenty pounds double their risk of heart diseases. Include fruits and vegetables in the daily diet. Limit the amount of salt, sugar, and high-fat food intake. Take advantage of meal programs such as Meals on Wheels, nutrition sites, and food banks. Contact the area agency on aging, state department of welfare, or the local senior center to sign up.

Poor eating habits may be the result of lack of money (look into food stamps), depression or disability, difficulty with grocery shopping and cooking, improper dental care, diminishing taste buds, and foods that cause stomach upsets.

Simple dehydration (loss of the body's water supply) can bring on mental confusion, disorientation, and other problems. Suggest drinking at least two pints of water daily, even if not feeling thirsty.

No smoking. Experts say health benefits can be realized no matter what age you quit smoking. Hospitals have support groups to help smokers kick the habit.

Limit alcohol intake. Drinking alcohol reduces life expectancy, causes nutritional deficiencies, contributes to physical disorders, and increases the risk of accidents. Seek professional help.

Review medications. Over-the-counter drugs and prescription drugs can be abused both by the elder and the doctor who prescribes them. See Managing Medications in Chapter Three, Emergency Preparedness, page 57.

Breathe. Use breathing as a technique for relaxation and to keep the oxygen flowing. Take long, deep breaths on a regular basis.

Use body products with caution. Understand labels on cosmetics, soaps, hair products, lotions, and deodorants. Buy small portions of a new product. Do patch skin tests. The terms "natural" and "fragrance-free" can be misleading. Do not share cosmetics, hair brushes, combs, toothbrushes, lotions, body sponges, face sponges, and undergarments.

Maintain a safe living environment. Physical changes in hearing, vision, and smelling affect comfort and safety. Get yearly eye and ear exams. Lack of smell may be a result of malnutrition or depression. Consult with medical professionals. See Chapter Eight, Safe and Secure, page 149.

Drive safely. Be realistic about the ability to maneuver an automobile on today's crowded, fast-paced streets. Nervousness and slower reaction-times contribute to deadly accidents. Wear seat belts. See Chapter Nine, Transportation, page 165.

Get a good night's sleep. Exercise, diet, and mental fitness contribute to rest and rejuvenation.

Maintain loving relationships. Companionship makes life more enjoyable and helps counteract depression. Spending time and talking problems over with those you are close to helps to overcome periods of depression, loneliness, and health problems. Family gatherings, social activities, church groups, volunteering, and sharing meal time provide opportunities of togetherness. See Chapter Twelve, Quality of Life, page 207.

Be informed. Examine the family's medical history at least as far back as grandparents to discern patterns of disease inheritance. Ask questions of family members and investigate medical documents. Keep current on medical discoveries and care options.

Practice preventive medicine. Get regular medical, dental, and eye checkups. Manage blood pressure.

Use medical services wisely. Find the right health-care professional to get proper care. Ask for referrals from trusted sources.

PLAN TWO
Know the health-care professionals and the services they provide.

All doctors are not the same. This list can help you sort out the differences and similarities among various fields:

M.D. (Medical Doctor) and **G.P. (General Practitioner)** are both physicians who treat diseases and injuries, do checkups, prescribe medicine, and perform minor surgery. They make referrals to specialists.

Board Certified Specialist, M.D. followed by, for instance, F.A.C.G. (Fellow of the American College of Gastroenterology), etc. If having an operation, check credentials F.A.C.S. (Fellow of the American College of Surgeons).

Internist, M.D. specializes in the diagnosis of disease of adults and its treatment.

D.O. (Doctor of Osteopathy) M.D. specializes in the medication and surgery of bones, muscles, and joints. Most osteopaths are family practitioners.

Any of the above doctors may refer patients to these specialists . . .

Cardiologist—heart and coronary artery specialist
Dermatologist—skin specialist
Endocrinologist—specializes in gland and hormone disorders
Gastroenterologist—stomach and digestive tract specialist
Gynecologist—specializes in the female reproductive system
Hematologist—blood specialist
Nephrologist—specializes in the function and diseases of the kidney
Neurologist—brain and nervous system specialist
Oncologist—cancer and tumor specialist
Ophthalmologist—eye specialist who also performs eye surgery
Orthopedist—treats and operates on bone, muscle, and joint disorders

Otolaryngologist—an ear, nose, and throat specialist

Proctologist—treats disorders of the anus and rectum

Pulmonary Specialist—treats disorders of the lung and chest

Radiologist—X-ray specialist

Rehabilitation Specialist—corrects stroke and injury disabilities

Rheumatologist—specializes in rheumatism and arthritis

Surgeon—treats diseases, injuries, and deformities by operating on the body

Urologist—specializes in urinary systems in both sexes and male reproductive systems

Mental Health . . .

Clinical Psychologist—not an M.D., may have obtained an academic Ph.D., specializes in family and one-on-one patient counseling

Psychiatrist—M.D. or D.O. trained in the diagnosis and treatment of patients for physical and emotional behavior disorders

Psychoanalyst—may or may not be M.D., treatment of patients for emotional disorders

M.F.C.C./L.C.S.W.—Marriage, Family, Child Counselor and Licensed Clinical Social Worker trained to diagnose and treat emotional disorders

Eye and Ear . . .

Optometrist—not an M.D., prescribes and adjusts glasses and contact lenses.

Optician—not an M.D., fills glasses and contact lenses prescriptions.

Audiologist—not an M.D., tests patients for hearing loss.

Dental . . .

Dentist—D.D.S. (Doctor of Dental Surgery) treats tooth decay and gum diseases, provides dentures, can detect mouth cancer, diabetes, and eating disorders

Endodontist—specializes in root canal

Periodontist—specializes in gum diseases

Oral Surgeon—performs difficult tooth removals and jaw surgery

Orthodontist— straightens teeth

Dental Hygienist—not an M.D., cleans and polishes teeth, teaches dental hygiene to patients, and takes X rays

Foot . . .

Podiatrist—D.P.M. (Doctor of Pediatric Medicine) diagnoses and treats injuries and diseases of the foot.

Additional health-care providers, many of whom are covered by insurance . . .

Acupuncturist—not an M.D., administers treatment by way of needles inserted into the skin and manipulated for several minutes. May be an Oriental Medical Doctor O.M.D.

Chiropractor—not an M.D., physically manipulates and adjusts the spinal column, joints, and soft tissues

Naturopath—practices holistic health care, including botanical medicine, manipulation, and homeopathy

Nurse Practitioner—N.P. registered nurses additionally trained to conduct physical exams, counsel, and treat patients

Licensed Practical Nurse—L.P.N. assists physicians and registered nurses

Occupational Therapist—O.T. provides individualized programs of mental and/or physical activity

Pharmacist—dispenses prescription medicines, knows about the chemical and correct use of medicines

Physical Therapist—P.T. restores mobility and strength to body parts affected by illness, disease, or injury

Physician's Assistant—P.A. takes medical histories, conducts physical exams, performs routine diagnostic procedures, and gives treatment plans

Registered Dietitian—R.D. specializes in dietary counseling

Registered Nurse—R.N. staff member of health facility or has private patients

Speech/Language Therapist—evaluates and treats speech impairments

PLAN THREE
Gently ease into action if your elder will not see a doctor.

A visit to the doctor can be a traumatic experience for the elderly. Use compassion to uncover their fears about health care:

• Ask your relative if he/she likes the doctor. If not, ask if switching to a different doctor is a desirable option.

- Suggest a less threatening health-care environment such as health fairs and drugstores where your elder can be tested for cholesterol and blood pressure.
- Older generations seek medical assistance in different ways than younger generations. Preventive health care is not typically a part of the elderly's thinking nor a part of Medicare, which is geared toward crisis, acute care.

Plan Four
Recognize that frequent panic attacks may be calls for attention.

On the opposite end of the spectrum, your aging family member may request too much assistance on a regular basis, making it very difficult for family caregivers to determine when help is really needed. Become an investigator. Enlist the help of health-care professionals and inform them of your relative's frequent requests pattern.

How to Communicate with the Doctor

In the past, patients believed that their well-being was solely in the hands of their doctor. Today, the best decisions that are made about health-care services, products, and methods of treatment are cooperative efforts between informed patients and their doctors. Even though this kind of doctor-patient relationship is healthy, most elderly people still feel reluctant to initiate conversations about a diagnosis or treatment.

In recent years, consumer groups fought and won the right for patients to expand their knowledge and options about health care. These changes help balance the relationship between doctors and patients and enhance treatment outcomes. Encourage aging family members to become active participants in their own health-care process, especially since compliance with the doctor's orders is a critical part of the medical treatment.

The more accurately your elder can describe symptoms and prioritize health concerns, the better the doctor can diagnose and treat his/her problem. Open communication depends on the willingness to ask questions. This may feel awkward at first. Health-care settings, with all the high-tech trimmings, can be intimidating; but putting in practice the action plans of this section of the planner—writing down questions, noting important changes in physical conditions, tracking the family's medical history, taking notes during appointments, keeping medical records, and seeking second opinions—will improve the quality of your relative's health care.

Sometimes, family members have different styles of coping with an illness. Some elderly patients who are sick want all the information they can get, while others just want to be told what to do. The decision to become an active partner in the health-care process is ultimately determined by the patient.

Difficulties in the doctor-caregiver relationship are an entirely different matter. The physician's focus is on the patient, not the family caregiver; and as a result, you may feel left out of the loop. There are steps you can take to bridge doctor–family caregiver relationship gaps. Discuss your degree of involvement with your elder. If you both agree that you are a partner in his/her health-care process, let the doctor know that you will be participating in all medical decisions. Most doctors will comply with your elder's consent.

HOW TO COMMUNICATE WITH THE DOCTOR

- On the average, physicians interrupt patients within seventeen seconds of the office visit and generally allow only eighteen seconds for patients to ask questions.
- Surveys reveal that the elderly are rarely told of the side effects of medications.
- The physician's role is also one of empowering patients to become active participants in their own health care.

The way the doctor talks and works with patients and family members is critical to the quality of the medical care. Some 70 percent of correct diagnoses depend solely on what patients tell their doctor.

Objectives

*After completing **How to Communicate with the Doctor** you will be able to:*

Gain a better understanding of your elder's attitude toward medical care.

Help elderly patients become intelligent consumers of medical services.

Enhance the quality of care your relative receives from health-care providers.

Help your elder to invoke his/her rights as a patient.

PLAN ONE
Be aware of your elder's attitude regarding medical attention.

Following are some health-care attitudes to watch out for. Your elder may:

- fear the truth and put off doctor visits based on what the doctor may say is the problem.
- not understand medical jargon and does not ask the doctor questions.
- be misinformed and prejudiced about aging and believe that the problem cannot be cured.
- maintain a death-wish attitude and may not be open-minded to any treatment.
- feel responsible for being ill and is angry with him/herself about being unhealthy.
- not trust health-care providers and does not believe what they say is true.
- have issues about privacy and senses a loss of dignity when anyone examines his/her body.
- be in awe of the doctor—he or she may hesitate to take up too much of the doctor's time and may be afraid to make the doctor mad.
- succumb to a false sense of security when the "experts" take over.
- rely on health-care providers for feedback on how his or her own body is functioning.
- think a good patient is someone who does not ask questions or challenge the doctor's opinion.

PLAN TWO
Know your elder's rights as a medical consumer.

Patients are entitled to:

- Privacy in treatment
- Be treated with dignity and respect
- Free, initial consultation interviews
- Informed, certified, properly trained practitioners
- Practitioners who meet timely scheduled appointments
- Be fully informed of medical condition
- Ask questions and participate in planning medical treatment

- Refuse treatment and understand consequences of such refusal
- Second or third opinions
- Prompt, clear explanations of test results
- Twenty-four-hour accessible medical services
- Refuse to participate in experimental research

PLAN THREE
Help your elder to become a smart health-care consumer.

Patients are better off when they learn to communicate with the doctor—your elder may be diagnosed more accurately, respond better to treatment, and recover more quickly. Helping your aging family members to implement the following action plans will help them feel more in control and tolerate symptoms better.

Before the doctor visit . . .

- **Put *everything* in writing.** Bring notes from home and take notes during the medical appointment. Bring a list of questions, health concerns, and symptoms, including when they started, times and patterns when they occur. Jot down any situations that are causing you stress.
- **Bring a medical history to *every* appointment.** (See Plan Four)
- **Attend *all* appointments with a family member.** No matter how routine the doctor visit, make arrangements for someone to be present to translate information, ask questions, take notes, provide comfort, and act as an advocate. Companions also help a patient recall what the doctor said.

During the doctor's visit . . .

- **Prioritize health concerns.** Start with the most important problem. Also let the doctor know about any stressful situations you may be experiencing at this time. When the doctor talks, write down explanations and instructions or use a small cassette recorder to tape the appointment and transcribe your notes later.
- **Ask questions.** There is no such thing as a silly question.
- **Understand answers.** Ask the doctor to define medical jargon, repeat things, refer to medical diagrams, and put information and instructions in writing. Keep asking questions until you fully understand what is being said and at the

end of the appointment, ask the doctor to summarize the visit to be certain important points are not missed.

• **Get copies of your medical tests** and ask someone to help you read them.

After the doctor's visit . . .

• **Get second opinions.** If you are unsure of what to do or do not agree with the method of treatment suggested, get a second and even a third opinion.
• **Manage drug prescriptions.** See Managing Medications in Chapter Three, Emergency Preparedness, page 57.
• **Stay informed.** Read, watch medical programs when televised, attend classes and health fairs.
• **Quality care is a two-way street.** Have the courtesy to call and cancel if you cannot make any doctor's appointments.

Shop around. Choose medical providers based on a satisfying relationship and the quality of care provided. Find a doctor who:

• Seeks the patient's opinion
• Explains how health can be improved with lifestyle changes
• Conducts thorough medical examinations
• Explains possible side effects of medication
• Takes a thorough medical history
• Does not keep patients waiting
• Encourages questions about health condition or treatment
• Does not rush through visits
• Cares about patient's emotional well-being
• Makes the patient feel at ease

PLAN FOUR
Help your elders take control of their medical history and records.

Encourage aging family members to become active participants in their own health care by creating a *written* medical history that is brought to every appointment. Thorough family medical histories result in better health care. Obtain a copy of your elder's medical history and distribute copies to other family members.

Include . . .

Medical History

Name/Maiden name
Date and place of birth
Blood type
Allergies
Past attending physicians and health-care providers
Current attending physicians and health-care providers
Pregnancies
Immunization records
Cause of illnesses and dates they occurred
Cause of accidents and dates they occurred
Operations and dates they were performed
Reason and dates of hospitalizations
Test lab results
Use of eyeglasses, hearing aid, walking devices
Negative reactions to past medical treatments
Successful reactions to past medical treatments
Existing health problems
Current changes in bodily functions
Personal stress and family problems
Insurance records
Mother's medical history
Mother's date and cause of death
Father's medical history
Father's date and cause of death
Grandparents' medical history
Grandparents' dates and causes of death

Medications History

Current use of medications:
   drug name
   drug purpose
   amount to take
   when to take
   how to take

how long to take
possible side effects
Current use of over-the-counter drugs
Current use of vitamins/supplements/herbs
History of drug side effects

Keeping total control of family medical records may be impossible but there are steps to take to ensure accuracy and privacy:

- Never sign a blanket authorization that does not specify usage.
- Ask the doctor who has access to the records and for what purpose.
- Review the records for accuracy, especially if they are sent to a health insurance carrier or life insurance company.

PLAN FIVE
Get involved by asking questions.

Your elder should have answers to the following questions *before* leaving the doctor's office.
The problem . . .

What is the exact diagnosis?
What caused this illness?
What is this illness called?
Will this illness go away, get worse, or recur?
Are there any likely medical complications?
Will the pain go away?
What lifestyle changes can I expect?
Can I see my medical chart?

The tests . . .

Why are these tests necessary?
What will they tell us that we don't already know?
How reliable are these tests?
Will the tests indicate the exact diagnosis?
Will the tests let me know what to expect in the future?

Will the results significantly alter any treatment plans?
What are the risks involved?
Will my medications affect test results?
What happens if I refuse or postpone this test?
What are the chances of inaccurate test results?
What is the test procedure?
How will the test feel?
How am I supposed to prepare for this test?
Will I need help getting home afterward?
When will the test results be ready?
Can test results be sent directly to me?
Am I to phone for the test results?

The treatment . . .

What is your experience in treating similar cases?
How will you treat this illness? Why?
What are the risk factors with this treatment?
What are alternate ways to treat this illness?
What are the risk factors with those treatments?
What is the time frame for the treatment?
Is a hospital stay necessary?
How long will I be sick?
How long before I see some improvement?
Will I fully recuperate?

The medications . . .

If medications are prescribed, see Managing Medications in Chapter Three, Emergency Preparedness, page 57.

The surgery . . .

If surgery is recommended, see If Your Elder Is Hospitalized in the Emergency Preparedness chapter of this planner, page 64.

The costs . . .

Do you accept Medicare assignments?
What is covered by Medicare?

What is covered by supplemental health insurance?
What costs are not covered by insurance?
How much can I expect to pay in the long run for treatment?
What are the costs of tests involved? Does insurance cover costs?

PLAN SIX
Prevent wasted doctor visits.

Before making a trip to the doctor's office, remind your relative to . . .

- Check and confirm the appointment time, date, and location.
- Verify that lab results are back from lab and have been analyzed.
- Confirm that the specialist received charts from referring physician.

PLAN SEVEN
Encourage second opinions when faced with a major medical decision.

Getting a second or even a third opinion does not necessarily mean you mistrust the physician's judgment. This course of action simply confirms an initial diagnosis. For referrals on obtaining second opinions, ask the existing health-care provider to recommend a doctor from a different practice or hospital. Or call the county medical association, a medical school, the health-care insurance company, and Medicare for referrals.
     Obtain a second opinion when . . .

- Treatment will irrevocably change patient's lifestyle.
- A surgical procedure is recommended.
- Radiation or chemotherapy is the treatment suggestion.
- The doctor orders a series of tests.
- Patient is unsatisfied with explanations regarding treatments.
- Patient feels uncomfortable with the doctor.

PLAN EIGHT
Check up on the doctor.

Thanks to consumer advocacy groups and new state laws, it is possible to investigate the certification and qualifications of medical personnel, as well as uncover malpractice suits, misconduct charges, Medicare fraud, and disciplinary actions taken against medical providers and facilities by the state, peers, or patients. To obtain such information, call the state medical licensing board or the attorney general's office.

Several states now require hospitals to provide data on procedures such as death rates and treatment complications. Hospital annual reports are becoming more common.

Patients can ask medical providers directly . . .

Have you ever been sued? For what?
What percentage of your patients die in the operating room?
Do you carry malpractice insurance?

To date, physicians are not required by law to reveal they have tested positive for the HIV virus.

Ask the doctor . . .

Do you have AIDS?
Do any members of your staff have AIDS?
Do any of the hospital surgery staff members have AIDS?
When was your last AIDS test?
Are you willing to put this information in writing?

Low Cost/Free Resources

The American Red Cross, in conjunction with AARP, sponsors a self-care course called **Staying Healthy after Fifty**. Contact AARP for details.

Contact the local offices of the **department of public health** and the **mental health department** for further assistance with health issues.

Local chapters of **specialized illness organizations** such as the Alzheimer's Association, American Cancer Society, American Diabetes Association, Arthritis Foundation, Parkinson's Disease Foundation, and the American Heart Association can be found in the white pages of the telephone book.

If a **dietitian** is not part of your elder's health-care team, a local hospital dietitian, a county home economist, or a home economics teacher may be able to provide consultation about proper eating habits.

Neighborhood emergency care clinics, hospital emergency rooms, and the **pharmacist** can answer general health-care questions if your elder's attending physician is not immediately available.

Hospitals and adult education centers offer basic **nursing-care programs** to family caregivers who are providing home health-care services for their relatives.

ORGANIZATIONS

American Chronic Pain Association
PO Box 850, Rocklin, CA 95677, (916) 632-0922

American Health Care Association
1201 L St., NW, Washington, DC 20005, (800) 321-0343, (202) 842-4444

American Medical Association
515 N. State St., Chicago, IL 60610, (312) 464-5000
Website *http://www.ama-assn.org*

American Psychiatric Association
1400 K St., NW, Washington, DC 20005, (202) 682-6000
Website *http://www.psych.org*

American Self-Help Clearinghouse
St. Claire's Riverside Medical Center, 25 Pocono Road, Denville, NJ 07834, (201) 625-7101

Center for Mental Health Services
Website *http://www.mentalhealth.org.tacenter*

Help for Incontinent People
PO Box 8310, Spartanburg, SC 29305, (800) 252-3337, (803) 579-7900

Joint Commission on Accreditation of Healthcare Organizations
One Renaissance Blvd., Oak Brook Terrace, IL 60181, (630) 916-5600
Website *http://www.jcaho.org*

Medicare Hotline
(800) 638-6833

National Health Information Hotline
(800) 336-4797

National Institutes of Health
9000 Rockville Pike, Bethesda, MD 20892, (301) 496-4000
Website *http://www.nih.gov*

National Institute on Aging Helpline
(800) 222-2225

National Women's Health Network
514 10th St., NW, Suite 400, Washington, DC 20004, (202) 347-1140

U.S. Department of Health and Human Services
PO Box 1133, Washington, DC 20013, (800) 336-4797
Website *http://www.os.dhhs.gov*

Action Checklist

TAKING CHARGE: HEALTHY LIVING TIPS	To Do By	Completed
Set health-care goals (Plan One) . . .		
short-term	_____	❏
long-term	_____	❏
Access health care professionals (Plan Two).	_____	❏
Have a plan if elder refuses to see doctor (Plan Three).	_____	❏
Discuss elder's health attitudes with (Plan Four) . . .		
family	_____	❏
doctor	_____	❏
Obtain emergency phone number of . . .		
doctors	_____	❏
dentist	_____	❏
pharmacist	_____	❏
nurse	_____	❏
hospital	_____	❏
medical center	_____	❏
Keep important phone numbers . . .		
at home	_____	❏
at work	_____	❏
in wallet/purse	_____	❏
Distribute phone numbers to key people.	_____	❏

HOW TO COMMUNICATE WITH THE DOCTOR

	To Do By	Completed
Be aware of elder's health attitudes (Plan One).	_____	❏
Review patient's rights (Plan Two).	_____	❏
Set communication goals with elder (Plan Three).	_____	❏
Plan for someone to accompany elder to all medical appointments.	_____	❏

Create medical history chart (Plan Four). _____ ❏

Research family medical history. _____ ❏

Distribute copies of medical history to family members. _____ ❏

Prepare for doctor's appointments . . .
   paper and pencil _____ ❏
   drug-usage chart _____ ❏
   medical history _____ ❏
   questions _____ ❏
   symptoms _____ ❏
   medical problems _____ ❏
   stressful events _____ ❏

Verify appointments in advance (Plan Six). _____ ❏

Get second opinion if needed (Plan Seven). _____ ❏

Check up on medical staff and facility (Plan Eight). _____ ❏

Switch doctors if unsatisfied. _____ ❏

Chapter 11

DEATH AND DYING

Death (and Life) Is a Matter of Attitude

Intellectually we know that the caregiving experience ends with the death of our elder. Emotionally, however, we have no way of preparing or predicting how we will accept and deal with this loss when the time comes. For some caregivers, the death of their aging family member may seem like a blessing, especially if their loved one suffered from the effects of ill health. Others may find the loss especially traumatic and profound.

At the turn of the century, death was recognized and treated as a familiar and expected event. Today, however, most of us are removed from the actual dying process and avoid even thinking about the subject. Ultimately, the remaining family members suffer when they are unprepared to handle unfinished family business, especially under emotionally distraught circumstances.

This section of the planner assists family members in handling the sensitive issues of death and dying with their aging relatives. Conversations regarding the right to die with dignity, funeral arrangements, distribution of property, and arranging for research and organ donations relieve the family from making such arrangements and decisions in a state of grief. At the same time, your elder may experience greater peace of mind by knowing that his/her final wishes will be carried out as planned.

DEATH (AND LIFE) IS A MATTER OF ATTITUDE

- Since the 1930s, we have moved death out of the home and into hospitals and funeral homes, underscoring the tendency to deny the facts of death.
- By the age of fifteen, media experts say, the average American has seen tens of thousands of television murders and has been exposed to war, famine, and holocaust in the daily news. At the same time we have been isolated from the actuality of death, and it has bred a habit of denial.
- Psychologists report that most people spend the better part of their lives coping with losses, past, present, or projected ones.

Encourage your elder to plan ahead for terminal illness and incapacity as a way to lessen the psychological burdens of an extended illness.

Objectives

After completing Death (and Life) Is a Matter of Attitude you will be able to:

Understand terminal illness eldercare options.

Assist your aging family member with funeral arrangements.

Locate documents for the collection of rights and benefits after death.

Seek sources of emotional support during periods of bereavement.

PLAN ONE
Support the right of the terminally ill to die with dignity.

Hospice is a philosophy of care that helps the terminally ill patient, no matter what age, to die at home or in a specialized facility. Hospice essentially transfers control of care to the patient and the patient's family and is typically available on a daily, twenty-four-hour basis. Care and concern for the total family are what makes such care different from traditional health care. Ask which hospice services are covered by Medicare.

For those patients who are receiving hospital medical care, the Federal Patient Self-Determination Act requires that all hospitals give registering patients information regarding their right to accept or decline any kind of medical treatment, including life support.

Patients at home or in medical or nursing institutions also can choose to wear an armband that directs staff not to resuscitate if he/she so wishes.

To find hospice programs and other alternative programs for the terminally ill patient contact the local hospital, the state hospice organization, the Visiting Nurses Association, and the area agency on aging.

PLAN TWO
Consider funeral arrangements ahead of time.

Advanced preparation for funeral arrangements takes the guesswork out of what family members think their elders may want and eases emotional and financial burdens. Ask your elder to spare survivors the uncertainty of funeral arrangements by making plans ahead of time. This information needs to be incorporated in a letter of instruction or as part of a prepaid funeral arrangement and needs to be available to the family at all times.

When the time comes, funeral directors will be instrumental in assisting family members with the details of the funeral, including writing the death notice. Be prepared to give your family member's full name, any nickname, maiden name, cause of death, age, names of survivors, lifetime accomplishments, educational background, and club memberships.

Discuss the following funeral options with your elder. Take notes and incorporate what is said as part of the letter of instruction in his/her will:

Funeral cost	Clergy
Wake or cremation	Religious services

Funeral home

Custom casket

Open or closed casket

Coffin enclosures

Hair, clothing, jewelry, glasses

Pallbearers

Flowers

Charitable donations

Music/Hymns/Soloists

Speakers/Readings

Video tribute

Cremation services

Disposal of ashes

Cultural rituals

Graveside services

Military honors services

Burial site

Family vault

Memorial marker/Inscription

Limousines/Coaches

Motor Escort

Flower car

Memorial record book

Family acknowledgment cards

Special requests

PLAN THREE

Investigate the cost of funerals.

Pay-in-advance funerals are becoming more common and those who consider this option should proceed with caution. Prepaid funeral arrangements vary according to whether they are funded by an individual trust, a state-regulated trust, an insurance policy, or an annuity contract. Some prepayment plans are guaranteed, provide for inflation, can be transferred if your elder moves, and involve little or no penalty for cancellation. Make sure you are well informed.

Under the Funeral Rule of 1984, the Federal Trade Commission developed regulations requiring funeral directors to provide family members with an itemized list of charges for services, facilities, and equipment. Take a look at a sample invoice as a way to calculate what costs are involved.

In the event that your aging relative dies while traveling, investigate whether or not he/she took out trip insurance offered by most airlines, cruise lines, and travel outfitters. This kind of insurance covers the costs of transporting the body back home, emergency travel expenses of family members, and medical care your elder may have received while traveling. If your elder is planning on a trip in the future, ask him/her to purchase trip insurance for this purpose.

PLAN FOUR
Prepare death notification lists.

One of the many tasks family members are expected to carry out upon the death of their relative is making telephone calls for the purpose of notifying family, friends, co-workers, and others. These calls are emotionally draining and knowing who to call ahead of time helps to lessen the impact.

Ask aging family members to make a list of whom to notify upon their death. Ask them to write down names, addresses and telephone numbers and how they know them. If this list-making task is too difficult or time consuming, ask your elder to photocopy his/her personal address book and put a star next to the names to call. Make copies of this notification list and distribute to family members. Include a copy of the list in the letters of instruction as part of his/her will. Ask your elder to keep the list as current as possible.

If a list is unavailable at the time of your relative's death, look for names and numbers in his/her personal address book. As you call people, ask them if there is anyone else who needs to be contacted and ask for their assistance in calling them in your behalf.

PLAN FIVE
Decide now for an organ donation and an autopsy.

People who are interested in advancing science through an autopsy or wish to make an organ donation must make such arrangements in advance. Contact organ banks, a hospital, a medical school, the Department of Motor Vehicles, and the area agency on aging for further information.

The reasons for performing an autopsy include:

- To pinpoint the exact cause of death
- To make research available to an aging population
- To identify genetic disorders
- To stop the spread of contagious disease
- To assist public health authorities in tracking death causes

PLAN SIX
Secure vital statistics.

In the event of death, family members will need to know the answers to the following information regarding your relative, especially when making funeral arrangements and settling financial affairs:

Full legal name and maiden name	Marital status
Current residence	Spouse name (maiden name)
Last residence	Heirs
Birth date	Father's name
Birthplace	Father's birthplace
Citizenship	Mother's maiden name
Social Security number	Mother's birthplace
Military record	Marriage date
Employment record	Divorce date
Employee number	

PLAN SEVEN
Compose an obituary.

In addition to a death notice, family members may wish to submit an obituary to local and national newspapers as well as to alumni, club, and job-related newsletters.

An obituary typically includes biographical information such as age, cause of death, family relations, schools attended, years graduated, degrees earned, religious affiliations, civic accomplishments, offices held, employment positions, club or union memberships, military record, hobbies and interests, special achievements, and awards.

If you are writing the obituary after your relative's death, ask his/her close friends, co-workers, and relatives to supply you with biographical details. If you can obtain a copy of your elder's resume, its contents will be very helpful for this purpose.

When submitting an obituary, include the name, address, and telephone number of a contact, visitation and funeral services days and times, and any charitable donations and special requests. If you are submitting a black-and-white photo of your family member, write your name and address on the back if you want the photo returned.

PLAN EIGHT
Procure the sources of your elder's income and savings.

In addition to property and possessions, what is left of your family member's income and savings will be distributed to heirs and beneficiaries after taxes and debts are paid. Funds will derive from cash-on-hand, checking and savings accounts, paychecks, company pensions, insurance policies, retirement savings, tax refunds, trusts, money owed, rental security deposits, Social Security, veteran and union death benefits.

To collect these funds, legal heirs and beneficiaries must contact each source directly. Use Chapter Thirteen, Documents Locator, page 229, as a guide to locate companies, institutions, individuals, and agencies that may owe your elder's estate money.

PLAN NINE
Gather the documents necessary to settle your elder's affairs.

Family members will need to obtain the following documentation to close out your relative's personal and business affairs:

Will	Power of attorney
Trusts	Marriage license
Letters of instruction	Divorce decree
Insurance policies	Military records
Social Security number	Property deeds and titles
Social Security benefits and	Loan papers
death benefits	Credit cards
Certified death certificate	Property rental contracts
Citizenship papers	Income tax records and returns
Birth certificate	Personal and business contracts
Company pension records	Vehicle titles
Bank records	Stocks and bonds certificates
Bank power of attorney	Valuables and collectibles receipts

Property and assets that are not removed from an estate through a will or trust, joint ownership, or beneficiary notices must undergo probate (the process of identifying and paying heirs, creditors, and determining taxes). This legal process can take six months or longer. Family members can designate a presumed heir to act as the administrator of the estate, otherwise the court will appoint an administrator. Contact an attorney to get proceedings started.

Banks and other financial institutions require heirs to obtain legal **letters of office** through an attorney if durable power of attorney was not secured with the bank while your relative was still alive.

Purchase at least ten certified copies of the **death certificate** for filing claims, transferring titles and securities, and collecting benefits. The family doctor, hospital, or the funeral director can obtain copies for you.

PLAN TEN
Look for clues to find elder's missing documents.

If you and your elder did not complete the Documents Locator chapter in this planner and you have limited knowledge of the existence of important papers, there are steps you can take to uncover missing documents:

- Review your elder's **personal address book** for names and telephone numbers of important people and places.
- Locate your elder's checkbook and savings book for **account numbers** and names of banking institutions. Read the check writing entries to find out where your elder has been spending money and to define sources of deposits.
- Review your elder's **bill-paying history** to uncover payment plans and refund sources.
- Call each of your elder's **credit card companies** to find out if your elder took out an insurance policy. Cancel the credit card if it will no longer be in use.
- Search through your elder's **storage areas** at home and at work to find papers and documents.
- Review the contents of your elder's **home safe and bank safe-deposit box.** If your elder did not make arrangements for you to have access to the safe-deposit box, the bank may refuse to open it. If this happens, ask the bank what they require for you to gain access.
- Contact your elder's **employers**, past and present, regarding company pensions, life insurance policies, retirement savings, and union memberships.
- If you believe that your elder had a **will** and you cannot find it, check the local probate court to see if a will was filed. You can also advertise in the classified

section of the local newspaper and local bar association publication to inquire about the existence of the will. If several months pass and no will is found, it is safe to assume that your elder died without one.

- If you think your elder carried life insurance and you do not know the name of the company, **life insurance policy search services** are available through the American Council of Life Insurance. See Low Cost/Free Resources of this chapter for the address information.
- You can apply for certified copies of **marriage licenses** and **divorce decrees** at the office of the county clerk where the license and divorce were issued.
- Copies of **death certificates** of relatives are available at the county recorder's office.
- If your elder was a **veteran** and you need a certificate of honorable discharge to collect benefits, you can write to the Department of Defense. See Low Cost/Free Resources of this chapter for address information.

PLAN ELEVEN
Tie up loose ends.

When the funeral services are over, and the legal distribution of property and assets is in progress, the fact of your family member's death slowly starts to sink in. This stage of the eldercare process is by far the most emotionally challenging. Though you are experiencing intense feelings of helplessness and sadness, remember there are still more responsibilities that require immediate attention.

Take as much time as you need to make decisions regarding your relative's personal belongings, such as clothes, an automobile, and favorite items. Come to a consensus with other family members on what to keep, what to give away, what to sell, and what to donate.
Other tasks include:

- Notify the post office of the death and provide a forward mailing address.
- Cancel credit cards.
- Cancel newspaper and magazine subscriptions.
- Cancel club and union memberships.
- Cancel insurance when properties are sold or transferred.
- Cancel utility services, telephone, and cable television.
- If elder rented an apartment or home, clean up and ask for the security deposit back plus any interest due.
- File a final tax return. Store past tax records.

- Transfer vehicle titles.
- Keep a balance in your elder's checking account to continue paying the mortgage, loans, taxes, lawyer and accountant fees, liability insurance, and utility bills out of the estate until assets are sold. *(Family members are under no obligation to pay the bills of the deceased out of their own pocket unless the bills are also in their name.)*
- Lock up any additional property such as vehicles or second homes to protect against accidents and claims against the estate until such property is sold.
- Send acknowledgment cards to those who sent flowers and donations. You are not obligated to send cards to everyone who sent sympathy cards or attended funeral services unless you want to.
- Keep notes and files on every transaction and decision you and other family members made regarding your elder's property and assets. You may be questioned later on and the notes can be used to back you up.

PLAN TWELVE
Encourage normal stages of grief.

Bereavement experts note that the stages of accepting the death of a loved one include shock and denial, bargaining for time, anger, depression, and acceptance. They conclude that these stages of completion do not necessarily follow any special order.

The grieving process varies among individuals. Here are some guidelines for encouraging normal grieving stages:

- Do not put a time restraint on your grieving period.
- Give yourself permission to cry and express deep feelings.
- Understand that grieving may be delayed due to settling the affairs of your elder's estate.
- Lacking an appetite or losing weight is normal.
- Periods of feeling helpless and despair are expected.
- Vivid dreams of the dead may occur.
- Feelings of guilt, regret, and anger directed at the one who died, God, the doctor, and other family members are common.

Watch for excessive behavior patterns:

- Poor self-care, not exercising, not eating right.
- Isolating, no outside contact with other people.

• Speaking of the dead in the present tense in ways that are not healthy.

• Severe depression, speaking of suicide, nonstop crying.

• Alcohol and drug abuse.

PLAN THIRTEEN
Make use of bereavement support resources.

Friends and family are an important source of strength during times of grief. Since the length of time it takes to overcome loss differs greatly with each individual, family members can also consider alternative resources of bereavement support.

Call upon the following people to help you during this time:

Hospital social worker	Clergy
Church group	Support group
Therapist	Bereavement counselor

Low Cost/Free Resources

Most hospitals have **professional counselors** who provide advice and moral support for family members of terminally ill patients.

Hospice services are available by contacting the Visiting Nurses Association, American Cancer Society, Hospice Association, and the hospital social services director.

If you think your aging family member had a life insurance policy and you don't know the name of the company, start your search by contacting the **American Council of Life Insurance**. This service is free. Send a self-addressed, stamped envelope and request a *policy search form* to American Council of Life Insurance, Missing Policy Search, PO Box 615, Riva, MD 21140-0615.

If your relative was a veteran and you need a certificate of honorable discharge to collect benefits write: **Department of Defense**, National Personnel Record Center, 9700 Page Boulevard, St. Louis, MO 63132.

The **Federal Trade Commission** regulates the funeral industry and provides free publications. Available on-line from the FTC ConsumerLine on website *http://www.ftc.gov.*

ORGANIZATIONS

Cemetery Consumer Service Council
PO Box 2028, Reston, VA 22090, (703) 391-8407

Choice in Dying, Inc.
200 Varick St., New York, NY 10014, (800) 989-9455
Website *http://www.choices.org*

Funeral and Memorial Societies of America
6900 Lost Lake Road, Egg Harbor, WI 54209, (414) 868-3136

Funeral Service Consumer Assistance Program
2250 E. Devon Ave., Suite 250, Des Plaines, IL 60018, (800) 662-7666

Grief Recovery Institute
8306 Wilshire Blvd., Suite 21A, Beverly Hills, CA 90211, (213) 650-1234
Website *http://www.tiesoft.net/gri/*

Hospice Association of America
519 C St., NE, Washington, DC 20002, (202) 546-4759

Hospice Hands
Website *http://gator.net/~jnash/hospice.html*

National Funeral Directors Association
11121 W. Oklahoma Ave., Milwaukee, WI 53227, (800) 228-6332

National Hospice Organization
1901 N. Moore St., Suite 901, Arlington, VA 22209, (800) 658-8898,
(703) 243-5900
Website *http://www.nho.org*

Widowed Persons Service
601 E St., NW, Washington, DC 20049, (202) 434-2260

Action Checklist

DEATH (AND LIFE) IS A MATTER OF ATTITUDE	To Do By	Completed
Review hospice options (Plan One).	_____	❑
Discuss funeral arrangements (Plan Two).	_____	❑
Cover funeral expenses (Plan Three).	_____	❑
Prepare death notices (Plan Four).	_____	❑
Plan for an autopsy or organ donation (Plan Five).	_____	❑
Prepare vital statistics (Plan Five).	_____	❑
Compose obituary (Plan Seven).	_____	❑
Gather estate income and savings (Plan Eight).	_____	❑
Collect documentation (Plan Nine).	_____	❑
Locate missing documents (Plan Ten).	_____	❑
Keep family members informed of . . .		
letters of instruction	_____	❑
legal documents	_____	❑
funeral arrangements	_____	❑
beneficiary documents	_____	❑
Read information on . . .		
hospice	_____	❑
funeral options	_____	❑
grieving	_____	❑

Chapter 12

QUALITY OF LIFE

What's Age For Anyway

The elderly are more unique from each other than any other age group. For example, there are seventy-year-old people who need the assistance of a cane to walk and others who run long-distance marathons. Everybody ages differently. In addition to genetics, the process of aging is largely determined by an accumulation of life experiences and belief systems. Consequently, some elderly people welcome new challenges, while others do not care for anything "different," preferring a familiar environment; some reach out to help those in need while others isolate themselves from the rest of the world.

People who are misinformed and prejudiced about aging stunt the possibility of being content in later years. Losing one's memory is not a natural part of growing old. In fact, speaking and writing ability improves after age fifty. The ability to interpret music and art improves with age and the best time to become a philosopher is around age eighty. There are many examples of people in our past who continuously enriched their lives as they aged. Benjamin Franklin helped to write the U.S. Constitution at eighty-one. Albert Schweitzer was running a hospital in Africa at eighty-nine. Coco Chanel was at the helm of her design firm at eighty-five. Giuseppe Verdi wrote the opera *Falstaff* in his late seventies. Golda Meir worked up to twenty hours a day in her late seventies. Helena Rubinstein led her company until age ninety-four. Winston Churchill wrote *History of the English-Speaking Peoples* at eighty-two. Pablo Picasso painted into his nineties.

At the very least, this section of the planner will help you encourage your aging family members to maintain their personal interests and to stay in touch with other people. The benefits of simple activities like taking a walk, reading a book to a child, and volunteering may be just what they need to feel good about themselves and others.

WHAT'S AGE FOR ANYWAY

- The elderly are as misinformed and prejudiced about aging as any other age group.
- Satisfied elderly people live enriched, active lives in spite of their aches and pains.
- The fear of dying is replaced by the fear of living too long.
- Aging family members don't want to be a burden. They think about suicide as a way to make things easier on everyone else.

It is likely that your aging family member has thought about death to some degree and may express a need to experience honest, intimate relationships with themselves and others before they die.

Objectives

*After completing **What's Age For Anyway** you will be able to:*

Offer activities that can enrich your aging family member's life.

Create special moments of togetherness with your aging relatives.

Notice any messages of depression and possibly suicide.

PLAN ONE
Add life to years, not years to life.

The telltale signs that your aging family member's mental and physical abilities are on the decline include an increased lack of interest in people and activities. Sometimes your elder's medications are at the root of the problem. Emotional issues, however, require specialized professional counseling. The more self-centered an aging relative becomes, the more problems develop, and that can affect the entire family.

Issues stifling your elder may include:

- Fear of death
- Fear of disability and dependency
- Fear of not being needed or useful
- Fear of losing mental agility
- Fear of loss of taking care of self
- Fear of living too long
- Fear of isolation, loneliness, sorrow

Aging is a normal, lifelong process that includes an accumulation of experience, wisdom, and judgment. The elderly have the advantage and opportunity to live with more purpose than in their youth. If your relative is stuck in a rut, perhaps asking the following questions will rekindle his/her zest for living a meaningful life.

What interests you?
Where can you get information on things that interest you?
What is important for you to do right now?
Which friendships can you create or maintain now?
Is there anything you would like to learn?
Where can you get instructions on what you want to learn?
Would you like to teach or volunteer?
Would you like to pursue any unfilled dreams?
Who is alone and lonely that you can visit?
Have you kept all your promises to others?
Have you restored any strained relationships?
Have you contacted everyone you want to see or talk with?
Is there anything you would like to do that you have not done?
Would it be helpful for you to talk with a professional counselor?

PLAN TWO
Suggest ways for your aging family members to stay in touch with themselves and others.

Lucky are the elderly who have time on their hands. Perhaps any one of these activities will cultivate a new interest . . .

Drawing and painting	Pottery making
Color by number books	Sewing and needlework
Knitting and crocheting	Journal writing
Creative writing	Story telling
Teaching	Playing musical instrument
Inventing	Singing and dancing
Acting and modeling	Caring for animals
Letter writing	Telephoning shut-ins
Cooking and baking	Reading
Baby-sitting	Volunteering
Taking a class	Learning computer systems
Learning foreign language	Games and puzzles
Traveling	Photography
Collecting stamps and coins	Church activities
Gardening and house plants	Concerts, art gallery, museum
Crafts and hobbies	Employment

PLAN THREE
Focus on quality travel services.

Travel outfitters and places of interest that cater to the special needs of the elderly can be found in the telephone directory yellow pages under . . .

Amusement	Auto Club
Bed and Breakfast	Boats—Charters
Campgrounds	Chamber of Commerce
Cruises	Guest Ranch
Historic Places	Hostels
Motels	Resorts

Retreat Facilities	River Trips
Sightseeing Tours	Ski Resorts
Tours—Operators	Travel Agencies

PLAN FOUR
Encourage your aging relative to learn something new.

The learning process never ends. Learning centers come in all shapes, sizes, and prices . . .

Community college	University
Adult education classes	Senior centers
Public library	Seminars
Lecturer	Elderhostel
Clubs	Semester at sea

PLAN FIVE
Ask relatives to share their talents, skills, and experience on the job.

Research indicates that the desire to feel useful, not income, is the number one reason older people seek work during retirement.

Employment opportunities for the elderly are plentiful. **The Equal Employment Opportunity Act** prohibits discrimination because of age, sex, marital status, race, nationality, or religion. A working status, however, does affect an individual's Social Security earnings and benefits. Before starting any job, seek advice at the Social Security office.

Job opportunities are listed in the classified section of the newspaper and with employment agencies.

Employment options . . .

Security guard	Salesperson
Maintenance work	Bookkeeper
Telephone surveys	Maid/Butler/Valet
House-sitting/Pet-sitting	Teacher
Baby-sitting	Day care
Companionship	Food preparation
Gardening	Restaurant host

Plant-sitting	Actor/Model
Hotel/Apartment doorkeeper	Concierge
Cashier	Parking lot attendant
Receptionist	Carpenter
Light housekeeping chores	Plumber
Office work	Mail house stuffer

PLAN SIX
Draw life from giving.

Elderly people have much to offer and are usually willing to share when invited to do so. Volunteering and teaching provide your aging family members ways to make new friends, stay connected, and make a positive impact in someone else's life.

Volunteer options are listed in the white pages under Volunteer and Voluntary Action Center and in the yellow pages under Social Services Organizations. The classified section of local community newspapers often publishes volunteer listings. The public library and the chamber of commerce are additional leads for volunteer opportunities.

Volunteer options:

Youth groups	Men's and women's organizations
Child day care	Adult day care centers
Special interest groups	Museums/Parks/Zoos Docents
Church groups	Community outreach programs
Schools	Libraries
Senior centers	Community centers
Theater groups	Animal shelters
Hospitals	Nursing homes
Family service agencies	Senior advocacy groups

PLAN SEVEN
Satisfy your elder's spiritual needs.

The desire to maintain spiritual and religious needs as a person ages is an unfailing source of support. Spiritual quests often provide meaning and direction and a clergy person is a invaluable resource who can offer your aging family members emotional support and spiritual guidance.

Your relative also might want to get involved in the many activities and services most congregations have to offer, including:

Counseling	Volunteering
Education	Bible study groups
Retreats	Choir
Socializing	Prayer groups

PLAN EIGHT
Watch for signs of suicidal behavior.

Studies reveal that most elderly people who attempt suicide fully intend to die. Failure to complete the act is usually a result of poor planning. Elderly males are currently the highest risk group for suicide.

Mental illness, loneliness, poverty, grief, pain, and severe depression are some of the reasons why older adults consider this violent act. Covert suicidal behaviors include starvation, terminating medical treatment, and mismanagement of drugs.

If you suspect that your elder is contemplating such action and repeats messages of despair and hopelessness, follow these guidelines:

- Contact the family doctor, the local hospital, or a law enforcement agency and tell them of your concerns.
- Ask your elder directly if he/she is intending to commit suicide. You will not be putting the idea in the elder's head. If he/she does not have these intentions, the response will be a firm "No!" and anything short of that should be considered a dangerous clue.
- The ability to share feelings with someone is your elder's first step in getting help. Suggest professional counseling.

Aging with a Disability

The Americans with Disabilities Act has virtually changed the lives of elderly people and others who live with disability and chronic illness. From employment opportunities to access to public programs and telecommunication relay services, anyone with a disability can pursue an active lifestyle if he or she chooses to do so. Medical advances also have been major forces in managing disabilities.

Understanding what our aging family members may be experiencing in the presence of a disability or chronic illness like arthritis or osteoporosis will help us cope with our own personal struggles as we care for them.

Caring for a relative who has a disability is an extremely tough job, one that requires an iron will, emotional and physical strength, and the patience of a saint. At the same time, care receivers often endure great emotional turmoil because the idea of their being a burden on someone else is devastating.

Managing the caregiving process under these highly demanding and interactive circumstances requires ongoing adaptations in your relative's home environment. This section of the planner will guide you in eliminating or minimizing psychological and physical risks that play an important role in their mastering basic, daily tasks. Disabled people who are in control of their immediate surroundings tend to lead more productive, independent, and satisfying lives.

AGING WITH A DISABILITY

- Aging with arthritis is the most common condition older people manage on a daily basis.
- The Americans with Disabilities Act gives every disabled person the right to a productive, independent, and satisfying life.

Most of the problems that family members encounter with their relative's disabilities can be handled with large doses of attitude adjustment.

Objectives

After completing Aging with a Disability you will be able to:

Separate disability facts from myth.

Help disabled relatives maintain their independence and a quality lifestyle.

Gain a healthy perspective on what life is like with a disability.

PLAN ONE
Dispel false assumptions about living with a physical disability.

The key issue when dealing with elders and physical disability is not the person's age but the duration of the disability. Age does not define the treatment of the disability—the illness defines the treatment.

Living with a disability is not necessarily one of living with sickness. The family's attitude toward their elder's disability will greatly influence the choices of treatment as well as their relative's quality of life.

If your aging family member is living with a disability, be aware of falsely labeling your elder as sick or unmotivated. Your elder—and anyone, for that matter—is the expert of his/her own body and family caregivers should remain as flexible as possible letting your relative advise you on what he/she needs.

One myth is that people in wheelchairs are sedentary. It takes enormous energy to sit in one position for several hours, let alone all day. Also, it takes great physical strength to move the chair. This helps explain why individuals in manual chairs may reject electrically driven chairs, seeing them as signs of failure, weakness, and giving in.

PLAN TWO
Keep ability in disability.

Separate your elder's medical problems from psychological problems—they may be two different goals:

- Maintain access to knowledgeable health professionals and educational resources. Find out what is correctable, treatable, and curable.
- Find a health-care provider who is willing to be open to new ideas.
- Eliminate any architectural barriers in your family member's home. Rearrange the immediate environment to enhance both physical and psychological needs. Independent living enhances your elder's ability to stay in control of his/her own life and minimizes eldercare responsibilities on the rest of the family.
- Allow your elder's feelings of sadness, anger, and resentment to surface. Stifling negative emotions may wear away at your elder's immune system. Suggest support groups.
- Acknowledge your elder's feats of accomplishment—however small. Achievements give meaning to the lives of those with disabilities.

• Find elderly role models who are successfully engaged in life in spite of the presence of pain or disability.

PLAN THREE
Adjust your attitude to get through tough times.

There will be times when caring for your family member will be overwhelming and extremely frustrating. Make sure you ask for and accept plenty of help from others. Then take a moment to look at life from your elder's perspective.
  Elders with a disability:

• Have psychological hurdles on top of physical disabilities
• Live with the silent messages that they don't belong
• Must find ways to feel productive while accepting assistance from
  other people
• Live with the physical evidence of a disability (canes, wheelchairs, walkers)
  in order to function
• May be living in constant pain
• Use more energy and take more time to do the same basic tasks as you
• Often experience feelings of loss and isolation
• Fear abandonment
• Increasingly worry about paying for medical bills
• Live in fear of losing even more control

Family Power

The experience of being a family caregiver to an elderly relative is certain to alter your life. In the midst of hectic schedules and physical distances between family members, studies strongly indicate that families are returning to the nest. The trend to reconnect with each other emotionally, physically, and spiritually also is evident in the rise in church attendance, grandparents raising grandchildren, the frequency of family reunions, and an increasing interest in the subject of genealogy.

The process of being a family unit is a simple one. Acknowledge each other's accomplishments, big and small, and learn to forgive and forget. The memory of being together as a family will remain with you for the rest of your life.

The preservation of family values and the documentation of stories and traditions largely depend on the family's willingness to do so. Too often, once-in-a-lifetime moments are lost forever because no one took photographs or recorded events in a journal. This section of the planner offers simple suggestions on how to empower every member of the family to preserve special family events and milestones like birthdays, graduations, and ceremonies. Even young children can participate when you hand them a camera and ask them to take pictures at family gatherings. In the long run, relationship bonds grow stronger and the spirit of the family is passed on to the next generation.

FAMILY POWER

- The family is still the strongest element in our society and cross-generation socializing is vital to all generations.
- Loneliness is a side effect of our technological society. Roles are no longer assigned and the aged are not included as part of the community.
- It is the family unit that maintains the quality of life, since the American society does not have a built-in system for this.

To make a family work takes cooperation, maturity, and acknowledgment of values and tradition. In turn, the family can offer a secure base that protects against the stresses of modern life.

Objectives

After completing Family Power you will be able to:

Gain power and protection in society through your family unit.

Preserve family traditions and history for future generations.

Create opportunities for your elder to contribute to the family.

Provide final compliments and farewell expressions of love.

PLAN ONE
Make time to make memories.

Here are a few activities that help keep memories alive:

Stay in touch. Telephone; write letters; exchange photographs and family videos; send postcards; visit each other; cook and eat meals together; shop together; create family parties and reunions; celebrate family achievements; record greetings, stories, and songs on tape and send them to each other; vacation together.

Acknowledge each other. Congratulate each other, compliment each other, send birthday and anniversary cards, share events and milestones, send report cards, send copies of awards and newspaper clippings, invite family members to plays and performances.

Make each other feel special. Ask and give small favors, ask for advice. Say please, thank you, and I'm sorry.

Fulfill promises. Let the family know they can rely on you and do those things you say you will do.

Forgive and forget. Be understanding and allow for family weaknesses, failures, mistakes, and illnesses. Stick up for each other in private and public.

Know your family history. Explore family traditions and cultural ties and teach them to the next generation. Share memories, search for family roots, and keep family records. Document family stories on video and cassette. Keep family possessions in the family.

Say I love you before it's too late.

PLAN TWO
Get to know you.

The methods of searching for your roots (genealogy) and the places you will look for clues will be as diverse as your family. Start by conducting interviews with the eldest members of the family. Create a list of questions to ask ahead of time. Write down the answers and use a tape recorder as a backup. Do not interrupt your elders when they are talking or they may lose their train of thought. There are plenty of books at the library on genealogy, reminiscing, and how to write your life's story.

Show elders old photographs. Ask them to tell you the names of the people in the picture, how they are related to the family, the date of the photo, where the picture was taken, and what they were doing at the time the picture was taken. Write down these answers.

If your elder has possession of antiques, collectibles, and old jewelry, ask him/her about the circumstances when the items were acquired. Very often, photos and possessions will jar your relative's memory to reveal a generous amount of fascinating family history.

Explore attics. Look for some of these objects to verify names, dates, and places of special family events: newspaper clippings, documents, letters, report cards, invitations, passports, autograph books, costumes, musical instruments, dolls, collections, toys, hats, diplomas, notebooks, diaries, yearbooks, scrapbooks, baby books, programs from plays or concerts, diplomas, trophies, paintings and artwork, maps, award certificates, photographs, and obituaries.

Search for family records such as birth and death certificates, marriage licenses, divorce decrees, citizenship papers, wills, deeds, and medical histories. Visit or write the state archives and public records office for birth and death certificates. A death certificate will tell you when and where the person was born. The birth record will name the parents. Documents can be obtained from the county clerk's office, state vital statistics bureaus, and state health departments.

PLAN THREE
Stay related.

Follow these suggestions to stay connected:

Take photographs. Make it a habit to take along a camera or video camera to capture family members and events on film. Put dates, names of places and people on the backs of photos. Ask other family members to exchange photos and add them to your photo album. Transfer home movies, photos, and slides to video and make duplications for everyone to see.

Draw a family tree. Create a chart that shows how family members are related.

Organize annual family reunions. Designate a reunion coordinator, decide on reunion format (one-day, weekend, picnic, formal, informal), pick a secretary to handle correspondence and a treasurer to collect funds and pay bills. The library has many books on family reunions.

Share stories and write them down. This exercise places enormous value on your elder's life and culture. Draw up a list of specific questions and have relatives fill in answers. Copy the finished pages into book form.

Give gifts of memories. Chronicle favorite family recipes, knit sweaters, crochet blankets, frame family works of art and needlepoint. Make sachets with flower petals from wedding bouquets. Reset jewelry into a contemporary setting and pass it down to the next generation.

Remember family traditions. Write them down. Practice them.

PLAN FOUR
Encourage intergenerational activities.

People today are living a lot longer due to medical advancements. Five-generation families are becoming more common. When kids and aging relatives get together, what our elders share with us provides a certain magic to life and family traditions. Children who spend time with aging family members benefit from preliminary insights into the aging process.

Community centers and senior centers typically offer intergenerational activities and child day care centers are always recruiting seniors to join in the fun.

PLAN FIVE
Redefine the role of grandparent.

If grandparents and grandchildren live a distance away from each other and frequent get-togethers are not possible, make the following suggestions to your elder as a way for them to stay connected:

Visit on video. Document stories, act out nursery rhymes, sing and dance, give a guided tour of your home or neighborhood, play a musical instrument, ask questions about school projects. Give grandchildren opportunities to remember voices and faces.

Exchange photo albums. Include pictures of family, friends, family pets, and places you have lived. Label each picture with a short description.

Write letters and encourage responses. Children love getting mail addressed to them. Put fun things inside the envelope like stamps, stickers, comic strips, drawings, photos, animal pictures, and bubble bath.

Record bedtime stories on cassette. Send the book and the tape along so the child can "be with" you at bedtime.

Initiate telephone calls. Make it a point for grandparents to know what is going on in their grandchildren's lives. Discuss school projects, recitals, sports, friends, and hobbies.

An increasing number of elderly people are finding themselves in the unplanned role of parent to their grandchildren. Alcohol and drug addiction on the part of the parents are common reasons for creating these unions. Across the country, grandparents raising grandchildren support groups are surfacing and helping elders to cope with the special challenges they face.

PLAN SIX
Encourage your elder to give back to the family.

There is little question that our elders are happier when they feel needed and respected within the family. Get them involved and active with the following activities:

Minor home repairs	Chores
Baby-sitting	House-sitting
Light business chores	Advice
Gardening	Light cooking and baking
Storytelling	Documenting family traditions and history
Sewing	Small errands

PLAN SEVEN
Know that a pet may play an important role in your relative's life.

Elderly people often transfer much of their love and attention to their pets as a way to deal with natural losses in their lives. Pets often fill a void left by the deaths of family members and friends and adult children who have lives of their own.

Though you may not share your aging family member's enthusiasm for his/her pet, it is important to be aware of your elder's emotional attachment to the animal. Pets provide companionship and make our elders feel needed. Playing with pets takes their mind off worries and health issues. Larger pets, like dogs, may make them feel more secure. Watching fish in an aquarium or stroking a cat or dog helps reduce stress and lower blood pressure. Studies completed in hospitals and nursing homes revealed that pets can help minimize depression.

Pets make no distinction between the sick and healthy, young or old. An animal's love is unconditional and a hearty tail wag can brighten anyone's day. If housing a live pet is not possible, give your aging family member a stuffed animal to adopt.

Low Cost/Free Resources

Locate **support groups** by contacting the local community center, senior center, and the hospital.

State bureau of tourism, state historical society, state parks, and **chamber of commerce** offices supply travelers free information and maps.

Computer software programs are available for those who are interested in composing a family tree.

Conduct an Internet World Wide Website search on the subject of **genealogy** to connect with a multitude of genealogy professionals.

Pet adoptions are usually free to senior citizens. Contact the humane society.

ORGANIZATIONS

Adopt a Grandparent Program
Mountain Light Center, PO Box 241, Taos, NM 87571

Aging Institute
HIP Building, Room 2367, University of Maryland, College Park, MD 20742,
(301) 405-2470

American Association of Retired Persons (AARP)
601 E St., NW, Washington, DC 20049, (202) 434-2277
Website *http://www.aarp.org*

Direct Link for the Disabled
PO Box 1036, Solvang, CA 93464, (805) 688-1603

Disability Resources on the Internet
Website *http://disability.com/cool.html*

Elderhostel
75 Federal St., Boston, MA 02110-1941, (617) 426-7788
Website *http://www.elderhostel.org*

Generations United
440 First St., NW, Suite 310, Washington, DC 20001, (202) 326-5271

Grandparent Information Center
601 E St., NW, Washington, DC 20049, (202) 434-2296

The Long Term Care Campaign
PO Box 27394, Washington, DC 20038, (202) 434-3744
E-mail: *hn6533@handsnet.org*

National Aging Information Center
500 E St., SW, Suite 910, Washington, DC 20024, (202) 554-9800, TTY
(202) 554-0571
Website *http://www.ageinfo.org/*

National Center for Women and Retirement Research
Long Island University, Southampton Campus, Southampton, NY 11968,
(800) 426-7386

National Council of Senior Citizens
1331 F St., NW, Suite 800, Washington, DC 20004, (202) 347-8800

National Institute on Aging Information Center
PO Box 8057, Gaithersburg, MD 20898, (800) 222-2225

National Library Service for the Blind and Physically Handicapped Hotline
(800) 424-9100

National Mental Health Association
1021 Prince Street, Alexandria, VA 22314-2971, (800) 969-6642

Retired and Senior Volunteer Program (RSVP)
1201 New York Ave., Washington, DC 20525, (800) 424-8867

Senior Com
Website *http://www.senior.com*

Senior Net
Website *http://www.seniornet.org*

Workplace Discrimination—Older Women's League
666 11th St., NW, Suite 700, Washington, DC 20001, (800) 825-3695

Action Checklist

WHAT'S AGE FOR ANYWAY	To Do By	Completed
Ask life-enriching questions (Plan One).	_____	❑
Encourage an active lifestyle (Plans Two through Six).	_____	❑
Satisfy spiritual quests (Plan Seven).	_____	❑
Seek professional advice (Plan Eight).	_____	❑
Your relative has access to a telephone.	_____	❑

Elder has information on . . .

	To Do By	Completed
special interests	_____	❑
travel	_____	❑
education	_____	❑
employment	_____	❑
volunteering	_____	❑

Locate . . .

	To Do By	Completed
community centers	_____	❑
senior centers	_____	❑
religious congregations	_____	❑
support groups	_____	❑

AGING WITH A DISABILITY	To Do By	Completed
Review facts and myths of disabilities (Plan One).	_____	❑

Elder maintains an independent lifestyle (Plan Two) . . .

	To Do By	Completed
medical goals	_____	❑
psychological goals	_____	❑
access to professionals	_____	❑
environment barriers removed	_____	❑
transferring issues	_____	❑
transportation issues	_____	❑
other role models	_____	❑

AGING WITH A DISABILITY	To Do By	Completed
Review your attitude about disability (Plan Three).	_____	❏
Informed of treatments and solutions to disability.	_____	❏

FAMILY POWER

	To Do By	Completed
Create goals to make memories (Plan One).	_____	❏
Research family history (Plan Two).	_____	❏
Document family events (Plan Three) . . .		
photo album	_____	❏
scrapbook	_____	❏
family tree	_____	❏
audio/video library	_____	❏
Generations are united (Plan Four).	_____	❏
Define role of grandparent (Plan Five).	_____	❏
Elder is giving back to the family (Plan Six).	_____	❏
Importance of relative's pet is understood (Plan Seven).	_____	❏
Read up on . . .		
genealogy	_____	❏
family reunions	_____	❏
grandparenting	_____	❏

Chapter 13

DOCUMENTS LOCATOR

Quick. *Where is your dad's birth certificate? Where does your mother keep the title to her house? Do your parents have a will? Who has power of attorney if they are incapacitated? Do your parents have supplemental health insurance? Does heart disease run in the family?*

The need to furnish legal documents, property titles, family medical histories, financial records, and other important papers is critical in the eldercare process. Completing the Documents Locator in advance will help you avoid the unnecessary trauma and expense of having to locate important information under already stressful emergency conditions. Taking the time now to fill in the Documents Locator with your aging relative will offer peace of mind since there may come a time in the future when your elder is not able to advise you on the answers.

The sooner you complete this section of the planner, the better. The content is extensive, so be realistic on figuring out how long this process will actually take to get the answers. Complete a small portion at a time. When you are finished, review the contents at least every six months for possible revisions and changes. Store the Documents Locator and original documents in a safe location that is accessible day and night, seven days a week. Make sure designated family members and advisors have copies of this information and related documents.

PERSONAL BANK ACCOUNTS

Account name/number _____

Names on account _____

Bank _____

Telephone _____

Type of account _____

Location of account documents _____

Is second signature _____

Has power of attorney _____

Account name/number _____

Other names on account _____

Bank _____

Telephone _____

Type of account _____

Location of account documents _____

Is second signature _____

Has power of attorney _____

PERSONAL LOAN

Name(s) on loan _____

Loan number _____

Bank _____

Telephone _____

Type of loan _____

Location of loan papers _____

INSTALLMENT LOANS

Name(s) on loan _____

Loan number _____

Bank _____

Telephone _____

Location of loan papers _____

Name(s) on loan _____

Loan number _____

Bank _____

Telephone _____

Location of loan papers _____

AUTOMATIC BILL PAYING

Name of store/service _____

Contact name _____

Telephone _____

Date payment deducted _____

Name of store/service _____

Contact name _____

Telephone _____

Date payment deducted _____

BUSINESS BANK ACCOUNT

Bank _____

Telephone _____

Location of account documents _____

Business name on account _____

Account number _____

Type of account _____

Is second signature _____

Has power of attorney _____

BUSINESS LOAN

Name(s) on loan _____

Loan number _____

Type of loan _____

Bank _____

Telephone _____

Location of loan papers _____

CREDIT UNION

Union name _____

Telephone _____

Name on account(s) _____

Type of account(s) _____

Account number(s) _____

Location of documents _____

FOREIGN BANK ACCOUNT

Name(s) on account _____

Account number _____

Type of account _____

Bank _____

Telephone _____

Location of account papers _____

COMPANY PENSION

Name on pension _____

Reference number _____

Dates of employment _____

Company name _____

Telephone _____

Location of pension papers _____

RETIREMENT ACCOUNTS

Name on account _____

Account reference number _____

Type of account _____

Bank _____

Telephone _____

Location of account documents _____

Name on account _____

Account reference number _____

Type of account _____

Bank _____

Telephone _____

Location of account documents _____

SAVINGS CERTIFICATES

Depositor _____

Certificate number _____

Bank _____

Telephone _____

Location of certificates _____

Depositor _____

Certificate number _____

Bank _____

Telephone _____

Location of certificates _____

SAVINGS BONDS

Bond held by _____

Type of bond _____

Bond series number _____

Location of bond _____

Bond held by _____

Type of bond _____

Bond series number _____

Location of bond _____

STOCKS CERTIFICATES

Stockholder(s) _____

Stock name _____

Stock number _____

Broker _____

Telephone _____

Location of stock documents _____

Stockholder(s) _____

Stock name _____

Stock number _____

Broker _____

Telephone _____

Location of stock documents _____

SAFE-DEPOSIT BOX

Box holder _____

Has access to box _____

Telephone number _____

Box number _____

Bank _____

Telephone _____

Key location _____

HOME SAFE

Has access to safe _____

Telephone _____

Location of combination or key _____

BUSINESS SAFE

Has access to safe _____

Telephone _____

Has access to safe _____

Telephone _____

Location of combination or key _____

ACCESS CODES

ATM machine _____

Voice mail _____

Debit cards _____

Bank-by-phone accounts _____

WILL

Will of _____

Attorney _____

Telephone _____

Location of original will papers _____

Has copies of will papers _____

Telephone _____

TRUST

Established by _____

Trust for _____

Attorney _____

Telephone _____

Location of original trust papers _____

Has copies of trust papers _____

Established by _____

Trust for _____

Attorney _____

Telephone _____

Location of original trust papers _____

Has copies of trust papers _____

LIVING WILL

Will of _____

Attorney _____

Telephone _____

Location of original living will _____

Has copies of living will _____

Telephone _____

DURABLE POWER OF ATTORNEY

Given to _____

Telephone _____

Attorney _____

Telephone _____

Location of original document _____

Has copy of papers _____

DURABLE POWER OF ATTORNEY FOR HEALTH CARE

Location of original document _____

Has copies of the document _____

Agent _____

Telephone _____

Agent _____
Telephone _____
Agent _____
Telephone _____

LETTERS OF INSTRUCTION

Written by _____
Has original documents _____
Telephone _____

FUNERAL INSTRUCTIONS

Arranged by _____
Funeral home _____
Telephone _____
Location of instruction papers _____

DONOR ARRANGEMENTS

Donor name _____
Donor bank _____
Telephone _____
Location of donor papers _____

AUTOPSY ARRANGEMENTS

Location of autopsy papers _____
Organization _____
Telephone _____

SOCIAL SECURITY

Name of beneficiary _____
Social Security number _____
Location of Social Security card _____

MILITARY DISCHARGE PAPERS

Veteran name _____

Veteran number _____

Discharge papers location _____

INCOME TAX RETURNS

Name of taxpayer _____

Tax identification number _____

Tax advisor _____

Telephone _____

Location of tax returns _____

PASSPORT

Name on passport _____

Passport number _____

Location of passport _____

DRIVER'S LICENSE

Name on license _____

License number _____

State license issued _____

License renewal date _____

CHARGE ACCOUNTS

Account name _____

Account number _____

Name on account _____

Location of card _____

Account name _____

Account number _____

Name on account _____

Location of card _____

Account name _____

Account number _____

Name on account _____

Location of card _____

MEDICARE

Name of insured _____

Claim number _____

MEDICARE HEALTH INSURANCE SUPPLEMENT

Name of insured _____

Contract number _____

Group number _____

Insurance company _____

Telephone _____

LIFE INSURANCE

Name on policy _____

Policy number _____

Insurance company _____

Insurance agent _____

Telephone _____

Location of policy _____

DISABILITY INSURANCE

Name on policy _____

Policy number _____

Insurance company _____

Insurance agent _____

Telephone _____

Location of policy _____

HOMEOWNER'S INSURANCE

Name on policy _____

Policy number _____

Insurance company _____

Insurance agent _____

Telephone _____

Location of policy _____

REAL ESTATE INVESTMENT INSURANCE

Name on policy _____

Policy number _____

Insurance company _____

Insurance agent _____

Telephone _____

Location of policy _____

RENTER'S INSURANCE

Name on policy _____

Policy number _____

Insurance company _____

Insurance agent _____

Telephone _____

Location of policy _____

BUSINESS INSURANCE

Name on policy _____

Policy number _____

Insurance company _____

Insurance agent _____

Telephone _____

Location of policy _____

LIABILITY INSURANCE

Name on policy _____

Policy number _____

Insurance company _____

Insurance agent _____

Telephone _____

Location of policy _____

VEHICLE INSURANCE

Policyholder _____

Vehicle insured _____

Policy number _____

Insurance company _____

Insurance agent _____

Telephone _____

Location of policy _____

Policyholder _____

Vehicle insured _____

Policy number _____

Insurance company _____

Insurance agent _____

Telephone _____

Location of policy _____

VALUABLES INSURANCE

Policyholder _____

Item insured _____

Policy number _____

Insurance company _____

Insurance agent _____

Telephone _____

Location of policy _____

VEHICLE OWNERSHIP

Vehicle _____

Make and model _____

Serial number _____

Where purchased _____

Telephone _____

Name on title _____

Location of title papers _____

Vehicle _____

Make and model _____

Serial number _____

Where purchased _____

Telephone _____

Name on title _____

Location of title papers _____

REAL ESTATE OWNERSHIP

Property address _____

Owner _____

Telephone _____

Co-owner _____

Telephone _____

Bank/Mortgage company _____

Telephone _____

Location of documents _____

CEMETERY PLOT

Owner _____

Plot intended for _____

Cemetery _____

Plot location _____

Telephone _____

Location of documents _____

MAGAZINE/NEWSPAPER SUBSCRIPTIONS

Name of publication _____

Sent to _____

Name of publication _____

Sent to _____

Name of publication _____

Sent to _____

CLUB MEMBERSHIPS

Organization _____

Telephone _____

Organization _____

Telephone _____

MEMBERSHIP CARDS

Account name _____

Account number _____

Name on account _____

Location of card _____

Account name _____

Account number _____

Name on account _____

Location of card _____

RELIGIOUS AFFILIATION

Name of church _____

Address _____

Clergy _____

Telephone _____

BAPTISM RECORDS

Baptismal name _____

Date of baptism _____

Church _____

Telephone _____

Baptism records location _____

BAR/BAT MITZVAH RECORD

Name _____

Date of Bar/Bat Mitzvah _____

Synagogue _____

Telephone _____

Records location _____

ITEMS IN STORAGE

Stored in name of _____

What is being stored _____

Storage company _____

Telephone _____

Location of storage documents _____

ITEM—REPAIRED/RESTORED/CLEANED

Item owner _____

Item description _____

Shop name _____

Telephone _____

Claim ticket location _____

ITEM BORROWED

Item description _____

Lent to _____

Telephone _____

ITEM ON ORDER

Ordered for _____

Item description _____

Order reference number _____

Shop name _____

Telephone _____

Expected order date _____

Location of paperwork _____

PERSONAL CONTRACT/AGREEMENT

Names on contract _____

Telephone _____

Nature of agreement _____

Location of paperwork _____

MEDICAL HISTORY

History of _____

Birth date _____

Location of records _____

BIRTH RECORD

Name at birth _____

Birth date _____

Place of birth _____

Birth certificate location _____

ADOPTION PAPERS

Adoption name _____

Adopted by _____

State of adoption _____

Adoption agency _____

Telephone _____

Location of paperwork _____

NATURALIZATION PAPERS

Citizen name _____

Place of naturalization _____

Location of papers _____

MARRIAGE LICENSE

Names on license _____

Marriage date _____

State license issued _____

License location _____

DIVORCE DECREE

Names on decree _____

Divorce date _____

State divorce granted _____

Decree location _____

SCHOOL RECORDS

Student name _____

School _____

School location _____

Telephone _____

Dates attended _____

Graduation date _____

Diploma location _____

Student name _____

School _____

School location _____

Telephone _____

Dates attended _____

Graduation date _____

Diploma location _____

EMPLOYMENT HISTORY

Employee name _____
Dates of employment _____
Company _____
Company address _____
Telephone _____

Employee name _____
Dates of employment _____
Company _____
Company address _____
Telephone _____

Employee name _____
Dates of employment _____
Company _____
Company address _____
Telephone _____

MOTHER'S HISTORY

Mother's name at birth _____
Birth date _____
Place of birth _____
Birth certificate location _____
Mother's name at death _____
Cause of death _____
Date of death _____
Burial location _____
Death certificate location _____

FATHER'S HISTORY

Father's name at birth _____

Birth date _____

Place of birth _____

Birth certificate location _____

Father's name at death _____

Cause of death _____

Date of death _____

Burial location _____

Death certificate location _____

HOME INVENTORY (FIXTURES, FURNITURE, EQUIPMENT, APPLIANCES)

Item description _____

Model number _____

Purchase price _____

Value of item today _____

Location of receipt _____

Location of warranty _____

Is promised to _____

PERSONAL ITEMS INVENTORY (CLOTHES, BOOKS, PHOTOS, MEMENTOS)

Item description _____

Purchase price _____

Value of item today _____

Location of receipt _____

Is promised to _____

VALUABLES INVENTORY (COLLECTIONS, JEWELRY, ARTWORK, ANTIQUES)

Item description _____

Serial number _____

Purchase price _____

Value of item today _____

Location of receipt _____

Is promised to _____

BUSINESS INVENTORY (FIXTURES, FURNITURE, EQUIPMENT, APPLIANCES)

Item description _____

Model number_____

Purchase price _____

Value of item today_____

Location of receipt _____

Location of warranty _____

Is promised to _____

PET HISTORY

Name of pet _____

Breed _____

Birth date _____

Sex _____

Animal hospital _____

Telephone _____

FAMILY PETS

Name of pet _____

Is promised to _____

Name of pet _____

Is promised to _____

Action Checklist

DOCUMENTS LOCATOR	To Do By	Completed
Complete the Documents Locator.	_____	❏
Locate and store original documents.	_____	❏
Make copies of original documents.	_____	❏
Maintain twenty-four-hour access to documents.	_____	❏
Keep in safe-deposit box . . .		
stock certificates	_____	❏
securities and bonds	_____	❏
certificates of deposit	_____	❏
titles to property and vehicles	_____	❏
deeds	_____	❏
bills of sale—major purchases and valuables	_____	❏
appraisals of property and valuables	_____	❏
retirement bank account records	_____	❏
company pension records	_____	❏
contracts and legal agreements	_____	❏
naturalization papers	_____	❏
Duplicate and distribute copies of the following documents to key family members and family attorney . . .		
Burial instructions/Letters of instruction	_____	❏
Durable power of attorney	_____	❏
Durable power of attorney for health care	_____	❏
Trusts/Living will	_____	❏
The Documents Locator	_____	❏
Keep in fireproof box at home . . .		
birth certificates	_____	❏
death certificates	_____	❏
marriage licenses	_____	❏

DOCUMENTS LOCATOR	To Do By	Completed
divorce decrees	_____	❏
financial records	_____	❏
passports	_____	❏
insurance policies	_____	❏
Wills	_____	❏
Letters of instruction	_____	❏
Durable power of attorney	_____	❏
Durable power of attorney for health care	_____	❏
military discharge papers	_____	❏
income tax returns for past seven years	_____	❏
property tax receipts	_____	❏
warranties	_____	❏
awards	_____	❏
education degrees	_____	❏
personal property inventory	_____	❏
property photos/videos	_____	❏
cemetery contracts	_____	❏

ELDERCARE GOALS CHART

The most effective goal setting is specific, realistic, and written.

GOALS   GOAL ACHIEVED

1. _____ ❏
2. _____ ❏
3. _____ ❏
4. _____ ❏

Prioritize and list what you need to do to accomplish each goal.

GOAL 1.	Completed	GOAL 2.	Completed
Call _____ ❏		Call _____ ❏	
_____ ❏		_____ ❏	
_____ ❏		_____ ❏	
Write_____ ❏		Write_____ ❏	
_____ ❏		_____ ❏	
_____ ❏		_____ ❏	
Meet _____ ❏		Meet _____ ❏	
_____ ❏		_____ ❏	
_____ ❏		_____ ❏	
Buy _____ ❏		Buy _____ ❏	
_____ ❏		_____ ❏	
_____ ❏		_____ ❏	
Read _____ ❏		Read _____ ❏	
_____ ❏		_____ ❏	
_____ ❏		_____ ❏	

GOAL 3.	Completed	GOAL 4.	Completed
Call _____ ❏		Call _____ ❏	
_____ ❏		_____ ❏	
_____ ❏		_____ ❏	
Write_____ ❏		Write_____ ❏	
_____ ❏		_____ ❏	
_____ ❏		_____ ❏	
Meet _____ ❏		Meet _____ ❏	
_____ ❏		_____ ❏	
_____ ❏		_____ ❏	
Buy _____ ❏		Buy _____ ❏	
_____ ❏		_____ ❏	
_____ ❏		_____ ❏	
Read _____ ❏		Read _____ ❏	
_____ ❏		_____ ❏	
_____ ❏		_____ ❏	

ORGANIZATIONS INDEX

Access Living, 310 S. Peoria St., Suite 201, Chicago, IL 60607, (312) 226-5900

Aging Institute, HHP Building, Room 2367, University of Maryland, College Park, MD 20742, (301) 405-2470

American Association of Retired Persons (AARP), 601 E St., NW, Washington, DC 20049, (202) 434-2277, (800) 424-3410

American Association for Continuity of Care, 638 Prospect Ave., Hartford, CT 06105, (203) 586-7525

American Association of Homes for the Aging, 901 E St., NW, Suite 500, Washington, DC 20004, (202) 783-2242, (800) 508-9442

American Automobile Association Foundation for Traffic Safety, 12600 Fair Lakes Circle, Fairfax, VA 22033, (703) AAA-6000

American Bar Association, 750 N. Lake Shore Drive, Chicago, IL 60611, (800) 285-2221, (312) 988-5000

American Chronic Pain Association, PO Box 850, Rocklin, CA 95677, (916) 632-0922

American Council of Life Insurance, 1001 Pennsylvania Ave., NW, Washington, DC 20004, (202) 624-2000

American Health Care Association, 1201 L St., NW, Washington, DC 20005, (800) 321-0343, (202) 842-4444

American Heart Association National Center and Stroke Connection, 7272 Greenville Ave., Dallas, TX 75231, (800) 242-8721, (800) 553-6321 (Stroke), (214) 373-6300

American Institute of Certified Public Accountants, 1211 Avenue of the Americas, New York, NY 10036, (800) 862-4272, (212) 596-6200

American Medical Association, 515 N. State St., Chicago, IL 60610, (312) 464-5000

American Psychiatric Association, 1400 K St., NW, Washington, DC 20005, (202) 682-6000

American Red Cross, 430 17th St., NW, Washington, DC 20006, (202) 737-8300

American Rehab, 1910 Association Dr., Suite 200, Reston, VA 22091, (703) 648-9300

American Self-Help Clearinghouse, St. Claire's Riverside Medical Center, 25 Pocono Road, Denville, NJ 07834, (201) 625-7101

American Society on Aging, 833 Market St., San Francisco, CA 94103, (415) 974-9600, (800) 537-9728

American Trauma Society, 8903 Presidential Parkway, Suite 512, Upper Marlboro, MD 20772, (800) 556-7890, (301) 420-4189

Assisted Living Facility Association of America, 9401 Lee Highway, Suite 402, Fairfax, VA 22031, (703) 691-8100

Association of Driver Educators for the Disabled, (608) 884-8833

Auto Safety Hotline, (800) 424-9393

Catholic Charities USA, 1731 King St., Alexandria, VA 22314, (703) 549-1390

Cemetery Consumer Service Council, PO Box 2028, Reston, VA 22090, (703) 391-8407

Center for the Study of Aging, 1331 H St., NW, Washington, DC 20005, (202) 737-4650, (800) 221-4272

Children of Aging Parents, 1609 Woodburne Road, Suite 302A, Levittown, PA 19057, (215) 945-6900, (800) 227-7294

Choice in Dying, Inc., 200 Varick St., New York, NY 10014, (800) 989-9455

Christmas in April, 1225 Eye St., NW, Washington, DC 20005, (202) 326-8268

Civilian Health and Medical Program of the Department of Veteran Affairs, PO Box 65023, Denver, CO 80222, (800) 733-8387

Close Up Program for Older Americans, 44 Canal Center Plaza, Alexandria, VA 22314, (800) 232-2000

Concerned Relatives of Nursing Home Patients, 3130 Mayfield Road, Suite 209 W, Cleveland Heights, OH 44118, (216) 321-0403

Council of Better Business Bureaus, Inc., 4200 Wilson Blvd., Suite 800, Arlington, VA 22203, (703) 276-0100

Eldercare Locator, (800) 677-1116

Elderhostel, 75 Federal St., Boston, MA 02110-1941, (617) 426-7788

Elder Support Network, PO Box 248, Kendall Park, NJ 08824, (800) 634-7346

Family Caregiver Alliance, 425 Bush St., Suite 500, San Francisco, CA 94108, (415) 434-3388, (800) 445-8106

Family Resource Service, 1400 Union Meeting Road, Suite 102, Blue Bell, PA 19422, (800) 847-5437

Funeral and Memorial Societies of America, 6900 Lost Lake Road, Egg Harbor, WI 54209, (414) 868-3136

Funeral Service Consumer Assistance Program, 2250 E. Devon Ave., Suite 250, Des Plaines, IL 60018, (800) 662-7666

Grandparent Information Center, 601 E St., NW, Washington, DC 20049, (202) 434-2296

Grief Recovery Institute, 8306 Wilshire Blvd., Suite 21A, Beverly Hills, CA 90211, (213) 650-1234

Health Insurance Association of America, 555 13th St., NW, Suite 600 East, Washington, DC 20004, (800) 635-1271

Help for Incontinent People, PO Box 8310, Spartanburg, SC 29305, (800) 252-3337, (803) 579-7900

Hospice Association of America, 519 C St., NE, Washington, DC 20002, (202) 546-4759

Institute of Certified Financial Planners, 7600 E. Eastman Ave., Suite 301, Denver, CO 80231, (800) 282-7526, (303) 751-7600

Insurance Information Institute, 1750 K St., NW, Suite 1101, Washington, DC 20006, (202) 833-1580

International Association for Financial Planning, 5775 Glenridge Dr., NE, Suite B-300, Atlanta, GA 30328, (800) 945-4237

Joint Commission on Accreditation of Healthcare Organizations, One Renaissance Blvd., Oak Brook Terrace, IL 60181, (708) 916-5600

Legal Counsel for the Elderly (AARP), PO Box 96474, Washington, DC 20090, (202) 434-2174

The Long Term Care Campaign, PO Box 27394, Washington, DC 20038, (202) 434-3744

Medicare Hotline, (800) 638-6833

National Adult Day Care Services Association, c/o National Council on the Aging, 409 Third St., SW, Suite 200, Washington, DC 20024, (202) 479-1200

National Academy of Elder Law Attorneys, 1604 N. Country Club Road, Tucson, AZ 85716, (520) 881-4005

National Aging Information Center, 500 E St., SW, Suite 910, Washington, DC 20024, (202) 554-9800, TTY (202) 554-0571

National Association for Hispanic Elderly, 3325 Wilshire Blvd., Suite 800, Los Angeles, CA 90010, (213) 487-1784

National Association for Home Care, 519 C St., NE, Washington, DC 20002, (202) 547-7424

National Association of Area Agencies on Aging, 1112 16th St., NW, Suite 100, Washington, DC 20036, (202) 296-8130

National Association of Insurance Commissioners, 120 W. 12th St., Suite 1100, Kansas City, MO 64105, (816) 842-3600

National Association of Personal Financial Advisors, 1130 W. Lake Cook Road, Suite 150, Buffalo Grove, IL 60089, (800) 366-2732, (847) 577-7722

National Association of Private Geriatric Case Managers, 1604 N. Country Club Road, Tucson, AZ 85716, (520) 881-8008

National Caucus and Center on the Black Aged, 1424 K St., NW, Suite 500, Washington, DC 20005, (202) 637-8400

National Center for Home Equity Conversion, 7373 147th St., West, Suite 115, Apple Valley, MN 55124, (612) 953-4474

National Center for State Long-Term Care Ombudsman Resources, 1225 I St., NW, Suite 725, Washington, DC 20005, (202) 898-2578

National Center on Elder Abuse, 810 First St., NE, Suite 500, Washington, DC 20002, (202) 682-2470

National Citizens Coalition for Nursing Home Reform, 1424 16th St., NW, Suite 202, Washington, DC 20002, (202) 332-2275

National Clearinghouse for Alcohol and Drug Information, (800) 729-6686

National Clearinghouse for Legal Services, 205 W. Monroe, Second Floor, Chicago, IL 60606, (312) 263-3830

National Committee to Preserve Social Security and Medicare, 2000 K St., NW, Suite 800, Washington, DC 20006, (202) 822-9459, (800) 966-1935

National Community Transportation Association of America, 1440 New York Ave., NW, Suite 440, Washington, DC 20005, (202) 628-1480

National Council Against Health Fraud, PO Box 33008, Kansas City, MO 64114

National Council of Senior Citizens, 1331 F St., NW, Suite 800, Washington, DC 20004, (202) 347-8800

National Council of Senior Citizens, Department of Public Affairs and Legislation, 1331 F St., NW, Washington, DC 20004, (202) 624-9535, (202) 624-9539

National Council on the Aging, 409 Third St., SW, Washington, DC 20024, (202) 479-1200, (800) 424-9046

National Eldercare Institute on Housing and Supportive Services, University of Southern California, Andrus Gerontology Center, Los Angeles, CA 90089, (310) 740-1364

National Federation of Interfaith Volunteer Caregivers, PO Box 1939, Kingston, NY 12402, (914) 331-1358, (800) 350-7438

National Foundation for Retirement Living, 184 Gloucester St., Annapolis, MD 21403, (800) 626-6767

National Fraud Information Center, PO Box 65868, Washington, DC 20035-5868, (800) 876-7060

National Funeral Directors Association, 11121 W. Oklahoma Ave., Milwaukee, WI 53227, (800) 228-6332

National Health Council, 1730 M St., NW, Suite 500, Washington, DC 20036, (202) 785-3910

National Health Information Hotline, (800) 336-4797

National Hispanic Council on Aging, 2713 Ontario Road, NW, Suite 200, Washington, DC 20009, (202) 265-1288

National Hospice Organization, 1901 N. Moore St., Suite 901, Arlington, VA 22209, (800) 658-8898, (703) 243-5900

National Indian Council on Aging, 6400 Uptown Blvd., NE, City Center, Suite 510-W, Albuquerque, NM 87110, (505) 888-3302

National Institutes of Health, 9000 Rockville Pike, Bethesda, MD 20892, (301) 496-4000

National Institute on Aging Helpline, (800) 222-2225

National Library Service for the Blind and Physically Handicapped Hotline, (800) 424-9100

National Meals on Wheels Foundation, 2675 44th St., SW, Suite 305, Grand Rapids, MI 49509, (616) 531-0090

National Mental Health Association, 1021 Prince Street, Alexandria, VA 22314-2971, (800) 969-6642

National Organization of Social Security Claimant's Representatives, 9 E. Central Ave., Pearl River, NY 10965, (914) 735-8812, (800) 431-2804

National Pacific/Asian Resource Center on Aging, Melbourne Tower, 1511 3rd St., Suite 914, Seattle, WA 98101, (206) 624-1221

National Safety Council, 1121 Spring Lake Dr., Itasca, IL 60143, (800) 621-7619

National Second Surgical Opinion Program, 330 Independence Ave., SW, Washington, DC 20201, (800) 638-6833, In MD (800) 492-5503

National Senior Citizen Law Center, 1815 H St., NW, Suite 700, Washington, DC 20006, (202) 887-5280

National Shared Housing Resource Center, 321 E. 25th St., Baltimore, MD 21218, (410) 235-4454

National Support Center for Families of the Aging, (215) 544-5933

National Women's Health Network, 514 10th St., NW, Suite 400, Washington, DC 20004, (202) 347-1140

Nursing Home Information Hotline, Washington, DC 20005, (202) 347-8800

Older Women's League, 666 11th St., NW, Suite 700, Washington, DC 20001, (202) 783-6686

Pension Rights Center, 918 16th St., NW, Suite 704, Washington, DC 20006, (202) 296-3776

Retired and Senior Volunteer Program (RSVP), 1201 New York Ave., Washington, DC 20525, (800) 424-8867

Social Security Administration, 6401 Security Blvd., Room 4J5, Baltimore, MD 21235, (800) 772-1213

U.S. Department of Health and Human Services, PO Box 1133, Washington, DC 20013, (800) 336-4797

Visiting Nurses Association of America, 3801 E. Florida, Suite 900, Denver, CO 80210, (888) 866-8773

Volunteers of America, Inc., 3939 N. Causeway Blvd., Suite 400, Meairie, LA 70002, (800) 899-0089, (504) 837-2652

Well Spouse Foundation, 610 Lexington Ave., Suite 814, New York, NY 10022, (800) 838-0879, (212) 644-1241

Widowed Persons Service, 601 E Street, NW, Washington, DC 20049, (202) 434-2260

Workplace Discrimination—Older Women's League, 666 11th St., NW, Suite 700, Washington, DC 20001, (800) 825-3695

WEBSITE INDEX

Administration on Aging's Directory of Web
Aging Sites
http:www.aoa.dhhs.gov/aoa/webres/craig.htm

American Association of Homes and Services
for the Aging
http://www.spry.org/aahsa.htm

American Association of Retired Persons
(AARP)
http://www.aarp.org

American Bar Association
http://www.abanet.org

American Medical Association
http://www.ama-assn.org

American Psychiatric Association
http://www.psych.org

American Red Cross
http://www.crossnet.org/triangle/otherarc.htm

Bureau of Elder and Adult Resource
Directory
http://www.state.me.us/beas/resource.htm

Catholic Charities USA
http://ccsj.org/links.html

Center for Mental Health Services
http://www.mentalhealth.org.tacenter

Choice in Dying, Inc.
http://www.choices.org

Community Transportation Association of
America
http://www.ctaa.org

Consumer Information Center
http://www.pueblo.gsa.gov

Council of Better Business Bureaus, Inc.
http://www.bbb.org/bbb

Disability Resources on the Internet
http://disability.com/cool.html

Elderhostel
http://www.elderhostel.org

Eldercare Web
http://www.ice.net/~kstevens/elderweb.htm

Federal Trade Commission
http://www.ftc.gov

Grief Recovery Institute
http://www.tiesoft.net/gri/

Health Care Financing Administration
(Medicare and Medicaid)
http://www.hcfa.gov

Hospice Hands
http://gator.net/~jnash/hospice.html

Insurance Information Institute
http://www.iii.org

International Association for Financial Planning
http://www.iafp.org

Joint Commission on Accreditation of Healthcare Organizations
http://www.jcaho.org

National Academy of Elder Law Attorneys
http://www.naela.com/elderlaw

National Aging Information Center
http://www.ageinfo.org/

National Association for Home Care
http://www.nahc.org/

National Association of Insurance Commissioners
http://www.naic.org

National Committee for Quality Assurance
http://www.ncqa.org

National Fraud Information Center
http://www.fraud.org

National Hospice Organization
http://www.nho.org

National Institutes of Health
http://www.nih.gov

National Senior Citizen Law Center
http://www.nscla.org

Senior Com
http://www.senior.com

Senior Net
http://www.seniornet.org

Senior Options
http://senioroptions.com/

Social Security Administration
http://www.ssa.gov

U.S. Department of Health and Human Services
http://www.os.dhhs.gov

U.S. Department of Housing and Urban Development (HUD)
http://hud/gov/senior.html.

The Wealth Center
http://www.aecnet.com/matters

SUBJECT INDEX

Access, 52–56
   checklist, 75–76
   code locator, 234
Accidents, 66, 69
Accountant, 70
Acupuncturist, 178
Address book, 54, 70, 198, 201
Adoption papers, 244
Adult day health care, 40, 73, 126
   finding, 47
Adult foster care, 138
Adult protection services, 162
Advocacy organizations, 146
Agencies, in-home help, 35–36, 38
Aging
   checklist, 227–28
   and disability, 214–24
   and quality of life, 207–13
AIDS, 189
Aid to Families with Dependent Children, 94
Alcohol, 63, 175
Allergies, 55, 56, 63
Alzheimer's disease, 45, 55, 127
Americans with Disabilities Act, 214, 215
Angina, 55
Appointments, 10, 70. *See also* Doctor
Area agency on aging, 40, 46, 93, 112, 127, 145, 170, 196
Arthritis, 45, 215
Assets, 82, 103, 104
Assisted-living facilities, 11, 137–38

Asthma, 55
Attitudes of elder
   and death and dying, 194–95
   and disability, 216–17
   and health-care, 182
   help needed with, 28
Audiologist, 177
Automobile, 241
   insurance, 89, 90, 118, 167, 240
   See also Driving
Autopsy, 198

Banking
   access, 54
   account locators, 230–32
   and death, 200–1
   finding accounts, 98, 201
   and hospitalization, 70, 71
   and power of attorney, 54, 106
   and safety, 156
   and transportation, 168
Baptism records, 243
Bar/Bat Mitzvah records, 243
Bedtime stories, 223
Behavioral health programs, 12
Benefits eligibility, 13, 93, 94
   checklist, 88
Bereavement support resources, 204
Bills, 70, 231
   payment history, 201
   reducing, 88–89

Birth records, 244
Blood type, 56
Board Certified Specialist, 176
Body products, 175
Braille TDDs, 74, 161
Breathing techniques, 175
Budget worksheet, 87
Burglary precautions, 89, 154–55
Business
   accounts, 231
   clubs, 21
   contacts, 67, 70–71
   insurance, 118, 239
   inventory, 248
   loans, 231
   safes, 234

Cancer, 45
Capitol hotline, 112
Cardiologist, 176
Caregiver, family, 26–51
   action plan, 49
   checklist, 49–51
   costs incurred by, 78, 80–81, 84
   and doctor, 180
   education for, 46
   elder living with, 142–44
   expenses of, 80–81
   getting helpers for, 33–34, 49
   help from family members, 45–46
   nursing-care education for, 190
   programs for, 40
   resources, 46–48
   self-care, 42–45, 51
   and sharing care, 31–41, 49–51
   stress, 44, 51
   support for, 12, 67
   task list, 19
   and telling when elder needs help, 26–30
Caregiver, paid, 49–51
   communicating with, 38
   hiring, 34–35, 37–38
   monitoring, 37–39
Caregiver, volunteer, 41
Carrier alert, 40, 74, 157

Cash reserve, 92
Cataracts, 55
Cemetery plot, 241
Certified Financial Planner (CFP), 83, 91
Charge accounts, 237–38
Checkbook, 201
Checking accounts, 54, 201, 203
Check-in systems, 52, 55, 76, 156–58
Chemotherapy, 188
Chiropractor, 178
Clinical psychologist, 177
Club memberships, 242
Cognitive problems, 28–29
Community Action Commissions (CAC), 22
Community programs, 12, 39–40, 50
   and financial help, 94
   finding, 21
   health fairs, 13
Companion services, 13–14
Computer
   on-line, 12, 21
   software for family tree, 224
Con artists, 158–61
Conservatorship, 107
Contact lenses, 55
Contracts, 20, 37, 244
Coronary bypass, 55
Costs
   checklist, 100–1
   funeral, 197
   questions for determining, 10
   and receipts, 66
   researching, 20
   See also Expenses; Finance and money matters
Counseling, and terminal illness, 204
County licensing offices, 39
CPR, 74, 162
Credit card companies, 201
Creditors, 70
Credit unions, 232

Death and dying, 194–206
   and attitudes, 194–95
   and autopsy, 198
   and bereavement support, 204

checklist, 206
documents, 200–2
funeral plans, 196–97
locating income and savings sources and, 200
notification lists, 198
obituary, 199
resources, 204–5
and stages of grief, 203–4
and suicidal behavior, 213
and terminally ill, 196
tying up loose ends, 202–3
vital statistics needed, 199
Death certificates, 201, 202
Debts, 88, 119
Deductibles, 118
Deferred payment loan, 95
Dehydration, 174
Dental specialists, 177
Dependent-care tax breaks, 97
Dermatologist, 176
Diabetes, 45, 55
Diet and eating habits, 174, 189
Dietitian, 178, 189
Disabilities, 214–24
    and attitudes, 216–17
    benefits, 93
    checklist, 227–28
    legal aspects of, 107–8
    resources, 224–26
    telephone discounts, 97
Disability insurance, 118, 119, 238
Distance caregiving
    expenses of, 79, 81, 100
    and safety, 149–60
Divorce decrees, 202, 245
Doctor, 180–89
    appointments, 183–84
    checklist, 192–93
    choosing, 184
    costs, 89
    directives to, 107
    and hospitalization, 68–69, 77
    and hospital release, 72
    if elder won't see, 178–79
    and long-term care insurance, 126

and medication, 59, 63
notes on, 183
preventing wasted visits, 188
qualifications of, 188–89
questions for, 183–84, 186–88, 189
referrals, 12
second opinion, 188
types, 176–78
Doctor of Osteopathy (D.O.), 176
Documents
    access, 55
    checklist, 249–51
    and hospitalization, 66
    legal, 52, 55
    locators, 55, 229–50
    missing, 201–2
    needed at death, 200–1
    originals, 10
    safety, 154
Driver's license, 56, 71, 237
Driving
    alternatives to, 168, 170
    checklist, 171
    decision to stop, 165
    legal steps and, 168
    safety, 155–56, 175
Drug-usage chart, 59–60, 62

ECHO housing, 137
Elder
    activities to cancel, 69–70
    budget worksheet for, 87
    cash checklist for, 101–2
    checking insurance coverage, 118–19
    communication problems with, 16
    and contacts list, 66–67
    and decision-making, 20
    and death notification list, 198
    discussing ready cash with, 85–96
    discussing funeral plans with, 196–97
    and emergency information, 5
    enlisting, in recognizing problem exists, 29–30
    fears of, 209
    finances of, and cost of care, 79
    getting to see doctor, 178–79

Elder (*cont.*)
  giving back to family, 223
  how to talk with, 9
  incapacity of, and legal affairs, 107–8
  job opportunities for, 96, 211–12
  learning opportunities for, 211
  moving and transition, 144–45
  negotiating about driving with, 167
  pet for, 224
  preventing isolation of, 169
  questions for, if hospitalized, 69
  questions for, to rekindle zest for life, 209
  safety precautions for, 153–56
  staying in touch, 210
  suicidal feelings of, 213
  telling when help is needed by, 26–30, 49
  travel services for, 210–11
  vital statistics needed, 199
  volunteering opportunities for, 212
Elder abuse, 150, 158, 162
Elder advocacy, 109–12
  checklist, 115
Eldercare
  costs and budget, 78–82
  goals chart, 251
  and government policy, 111–12
  locator, 47
  savings and checking accounts for, 83
Elderhostel, 225
Elections and voting, 112, 115
Electric company, 162
E-mail, 54
Emergencies, 17–20, 24–25
  and access, 52–55
  check-in system, 55
  checklist, 24–25, 75–77
  fund for, 86, 90
  getting caught off guard, 17–20
  and hospitalization, 64–73
  medical alert system, 55
  and medications, 57–63
  packing for, 90
  preparedness plans, 52–77
  resources, 73–74

  and telephone numbers, 38, 50, 52, 75–76
  vital information needed, 56
Emergency response devices, 15, 39, 157
Emphysema, 55
Employers
  and documents, 201
  getting help from, 45
  and health insurance, 124
Employment history, 246
Endocrinologist, 176
Endodontist, 177
Epilepsy, 55
Estate
  paying bills until settled, 203
  reimbursement from, 83, 84
Estate liquidator professional, 92
Estate planning, 103–8
  basic terms and options, 105–6
  checklist, 114
  and documents covering disability, 107–8
  and giving things away early, 106
  and lawyer, 106
  making instructions known, 108
Executor, 105
Exercise, 174
Expenses
  elder's monthly, 80, 87
  help from family with, 95
  reducing elder's, 88–89, 101
  tracking, 70
Experts, 19, 20, 25, 34–35
Eye and ear specialists, 177

Falls, avoiding, 63
Family
  activities with, 175
  and asking elder to live with you, 143–44
  asking for help from, 46
  asking for time and money from, 83–84
  and caregiver stress, 44
  checklist, 228
  discussions with, 20
  and document copies, 229, 249
  elder activities for, 223–24

and eldercare expense plan, 83–84
and elder's medical history, 184–85
emergency phone list for, 54
empowering, 218–23
and estate planning instructions, 108
getting relief from, 45
gifts of money from, 95
and hospitalization, 69–70
medical history, 175
meetings and conversations with, and care
    gap, 45–46, 51
and pets, 224
and receipts, 66
reunions, 222
and role of grandparent, 222–23
roots and traditions, 220–22
sharing care with, 34
task lists for, 33–34
tree, 221–22, 224
Family Caregiver Alliance, 47
Family counselor, 112
Family service agencies, 22, 46, 112
Father's history, 247
Fears, 209
Federal Patient Self-Determination Act, 196
Federal unemployment tax (FUTA), 37
Financial adviser, 91
Financial and money matters, 78–102
    and access to accounts, 52, 76
    checklist, 100–2
    cost of caring, 78–84
    deposits, 20
    determining how much you can afford, 82
    determining who pays, 83
    documents needed at death, 200–1
    emotions and, 96
    family plan for, 83–84
    finding ready cash, 85–96
    and food, 79
    fraud and con artists, 158–61
    funeral costs, 119, 197
    income and savings sources, 200
    and living arrangements, 141–42
    and moving, 145

and power of attorney, 106
    questions to ask about medical expenses,
        187–88
    resources, 93–94, 97–99
    See also Banks; Costs; Expenses; Health
        insurance; Insurance; Taxes
Financial planner, 91, 97, 98
Fire department, 54, 74, 162
First aid instruction, 74
Food and Drug Administration (FDA),
    58
Food banks, 174
Food costs, 79
Food stamps, 12, 174
Foreign language services, 13
Fraud, 150, 158–61
Friendly visitor programs, 158
Friends, 69, 175
Funeral, 194, 196–97, 236
    costs, 119, 197
    resources, 204

Garage sale, 92
Gas company, 162
Gastroenterologist, 176
Genealogy, 220–21, 224
General relief, 93
Generic drugs, 63
Geriatric case manager, 20, 34, 48
Gifts, 95, 96
Glaucoma, 55
Goal setting, 8
Government
    agencies, 12, 46
    policies, 110
    See also State agencies
Grandchildren, 94, 222–23
Grief, stages of, 203–4
Group health insurance, 124
Group homes, 138
Gynecologist, 176

Health and medical matters, 172–93
    being smart consumer, 183–84

Health and medical matters (*cont.*)
  checking doctor qualification, 188–89
  checklist, 192–93
  communicating with doctor, 179–81
  elder's attitudes about, 182
  elder's rights and, 182–83
  fraud, 161
  getting elder to see doctor, 178–79
  and healthy habits, 172, 174–76
  and medical records, 184–86
  questions to ask doctor, 77, 186–88
  reducing costs, 88–89
  resources, 189–91
  telling when elder needs help with, 28
  types of health professionals, 176–78
  See also Doctor; Hospital; Health insurance;
    Long-term care; Medical history;
    Medication and prescriptions
Health insurance
  checklist, 130
  counseling, 127
  and home care, 38
  and long-term care, 125–27
  Medigap, Medicare, and Medicaid, 121–27
  and medical records, 186
  options defined, 123–24
  proof of, 66, 70
  questions for doctor about, 187–88
  reducing costs, 89
  safeguards, 124–25
Health Maintenance Organizations (HMOs), 38,
    124–25, 128
Hearing problems, 97, 175
Heart disease, 45, 55
Helper's list, 19, 24, 33–34
Hematologist, 176
Hemodialysis, 55
Hemophilia, 55
Hepatitis, 55
Home
  expense list, 80, 81
  inventory, 247
  management, 67, 70, 71
  medical equipment for, 12

  repair and maintenance, 13
  safe in, 201, 234
  safety, 161, 162, 175
Homebound elders, 22
Home-care
  expense list, 81
  finding paid help for, 34–36
  after hospitalization, 69, 73
  insurance and, 38, 125
  resources, 15, 20
  sharing care, 33
Home health-care agencies, 40
Homemaker services, 13, 33, 73
Home-nursing programs for caregivers, 46
Homeowner, 93
  cash from house, 94–95
  insurance, 89, 90, 118, 239
Home respiratory services, 12
Hospice care, 12, 15, 196, 204
Hospital, 64–73
  being proactive, 66
  bills, 89
  business to do, 70–71
  calls to make about, 69–70
  checklist, 77
  elder contacts list, 66–67
  emergency rooms, 190
  information from, 11, 12
  items for elder, 71–72
  length of stay, 65
  patient representative, 39, 73
  questions for doctors and nurses, 68–69, 72
  record-keeping for, 66–67, 77
  release, 68–69, 72–73
  social services director, 107, 112
Hospital discharge planner, 20, 45, 145, 170
  how to get, 20, 21
  questions for, 72
Hotline numbers, 12
Housing, 131–48
  asking elder to move in with you, 142–44
  checklist, 148
  determining need for change, 134
  and finances, 141–42

after hospitalization, 72
improving, vs. moving, 134–37
and moving, 144–45
options defined, 137–38
questions to ask about facility, 139–42
resources, 14–15, 138, 145–46
shared, 144
Hygiene, 28
Hypertension, 55
Hyperthermia, 55
Hypoglycemia, 55

Identification bracelets, 63
Illness organizations, 189
Implants, 55
Incapacity, 107–8
Income, 87, 101, 200
Individual Practice Associations (IPAs), 124
Information
    and decisions, 20, 25
    and experts, 20
    how to gather, 9–11, 20, 24
    keeping copies of vital, 56
    and medications, 59–60
    organizing, 9, 19, 24
    questions to ask, 10–11
    recording, 9, 10, 19
    who to call for, 11–15
    See also Notes; Resources and websites
Infusion services, 12
Insurance, 116–30
    advisers, 118
    agent, 70, 116, 118, 126
    bills, 124
    checklist, 129–30
    company rating, 119–20, 127
    and eldercare expenses, 84
    and hospitalization, 69
    life, 116–20
    locator, 238–39
    health, 121–27, 130
    and paid care providers, 38
    proof of, 56
    receipts for, 66

reducing costs, 89–90
resources, 127–28
See also specific types
Intergenerational activities, 222
Intermediate care facilities, 138
International resources, 13
Internist, 176
Inventory, 119, 247
Investments, 92
IRS, 38, 97
Isolation, 28, 169

Job opportunities, 96, 211–12
Joint-ownership, 103

Keys, 52, 54, 71, 76, 156

Lawyer, 70, 83, 91, 97, 106
Learning opportunities, 211
Legal guardian, 107
Legal matters, 103–15
    checklist, 114–15
    and driving, 168
    and elder advocacy, 109–11
    and estate planning, 103–8
    resources, 20, 112–13
    and will, 106
    See also Documents; Estate; Lawyer; Living
        will; Power of attorney; Will
Letter of instruction, 105, 236
Letters of office, 201
Letter writing, 223
Liabilities, 82
Liability insurance locator, 240
Licensed practical nurse (LPN), 178
Life-care communities, 138, 142
Life insurance, 118, 119, 238
    cash through, 94
    finding, 202, 204
    and medical records, 186
Life tenancy agreement, 94
List making, 19
Living trust, 105
Living will, 66, 107–8, 235

Loans, 96, 230–32
Lodging costs, 79
Loneliness, 219
Long-term care
    and insurance, 83, 125–27
    and Medicare and Medicaid, 78, 122
    ombudsman, 39, 112, 145

Magazine subscription, 242
Mail, 70, 71, 157, 159. *See also* Carrier alert
Marriage licenses, 202
Mayor's office, 21
Meals programs, 13, 39, 48, 174
Medicaid, 12, 98
    eligibility and benefits, 78, 123–24, 127, 128
    and spending into poverty, 83, 97, 125
Medical alert system, 55, 76
Medical chart, 66
Medical conditions information, 56
Medical history, 183, 184–86, 244
Medical records, 89, 186
Medical tests, 184, 186–87, 188
Medicare, 12, 98, 99, 238
    eligibility and benefits, 78, 122–23, 127,
        128
    HMOs, 124–25
    and home-care, 38
    Hotline, 99, 128
    insurance beyond, 121–27
    and long-term illness, 86
    and preventive care, 179
Medication and prescriptions
    chart, 60
    checklist, 76
    containers and labels, 62, 63
    and driving, 168
    free, 98
    and health habits, 175
    and hospitalization, 71
    improper taking, 61–62
    information on, 56
    managing, 57–63, 184–86
    monitoring, 59–60
    reducing costs, 88–89
    safety precautions, 62–63

side effects, 181
    why elder doesn't take, 60–61
Medigap policies, 121, 122–24, 238
Membership cards, 242
Memories, making, 220–21, 222
Memory loss, 207
Mental health professionals, 177
M.F.C.C./L.C.S.W., 177
Military discharge paper, 204, 237
Mother's history, 246
Moving, 144–45

Naturalization papers, 245
Naturopath, 178
Neglect, recognizing, 28–29
Neighborhood
    emergency care clinics, 190
    watch programs, 162
Neighbors, 70
Nephrologist, 176
Neurologist, 176
Newspapers, 71, 242
Notes, taking, 10
    and death, 203
    and doctor visits and bills, 89
    and health care, 183–84
    and hospitalization, 66
Nurse, 63, 68–69, 178
    advice, 12
Nurse Practitioner, 178
Nurse's aide, 73
Nursing care, 12, 119
Nursing homes, 119
    alternatives to, 131
    costs, 78, 83
    decision to opt for, 131–32
    and Medicare, 125
    ombudsman for, 39
    resident advocates, 146
    types, 138

Obituary, 199
Observation programs, 14
Occupational therapist, 178
Ombudsman, 39, 139, 158

Oncologist, 176
Ophthalmologist, 176
Optician, 177
Optometrist, 177
Oral surgeon, 177
Organ donations, 55, 194, 198, 236
Orthodontist, 177
Orthopedist, 176
Osteoarthritis, 55
Osteoporosis, 55
Otolaryngolgist, 177
Over-the-counter drugs, 57, 63

Pacemaker, 55
Packing, 144–45
Panic attacks, 179
Passports, 237
Patient representatives, 39
Pension, 232
Periodontist, 177
Personal care, 12, 33, 73
Pets, 224, 248
Pharmacist, 59, 61, 178, 190
Photographs, 221, 223
Physical therapist, 178
Physician's Assistant (P.A.), 178
Planning, 5–25
    basic principles, 8–9
    checklist, 17, 23–25
    getting started, 5–16, 23
    resources, 21–22
    when caught off-guard, 17–20
Podiatrist, 178
Police department, 54, 162
Possessions, 106, 243–44, 247–48
    and family history, 221
    and insurance, 118
Posthospital recovery contacts, 67
Power of attorney, 56, 235
    and banks, 54
    and death, 201
    durable, 66, 105–6, 107
Power of attorney for health care, 56, 235–36
    durable, 66, 107
    free copies of, 112

Preferred Provider Organizations (PPOs), 124
Preventive medicine, 176, 179
Prioritizing, 11
Probate, 119, 201
Proctologist, 177
Property, access to, 55
Psychiatrist, 177
Psychoanalyst, 177
Public housing, 138
Public library, 21
Public transportation, 169
Pulmonary specialist, 177

Qualified Medicare Beneficiaries (QMB),
    123
Quality of life, 207–28
    activities list, 210
    and aging, 207–13
    checklist, 227–28
    and disability, 214–17
    and family power, 218–23
    and hospital release, 73
    and interests, 209
    and job opportunities, 211–12
    and learning, 211
    and pet, 224
    resources, 224–26
    and sharing care, 33
    and spiritual activities, 212–13 and suicidal
        behavior, 213
    and travel, 210–11
    and volunteer work, 212

Radiation, 188
Radiologist, 177
Real estate, 239, 241
Recordkeeping
    and hospitalization, 66, 70–71
    and paid care providers, 38
    and planning, 9, **23**
    and receipts, 84
    See also Information; Notes
References, checking, 35, 36
Referrals, 40
Rehabilitation specialist, 177

Religious groups, 12, 70, 242
    information from, 12
    and quality of life, 212–13
    and volunteer services, 21
Renter's assistance, 93
Renter's insurance, 239
Representatives, 112
Research, 9, 20
Residential care facilities, 39
Resources, organizations and websites
    caregiver help, 46–48
    death and dying, 204–5
    emergency, 19, 74
    financial, 97–99
    finding, in telephone book, 11–13
    genealogy, 224
    health, 189–91
    housing, 145–47
    insurance, 127–28
    legal, 112–13
    paid care-provider, 34–35
    planning, 21–22
    quality of life, 224–26
    safety, 161–62
    transportation, 170
Respite care, 15, 40, 126
Retirement account, 232
Retirement facility, 137, 139–42
Reverse mortgage, 95
Rheumatologist, 177
Rights, elder, 65, 182–83, 196

Safe deposit box, 119, 201, 234, 249
    and death, 106
    finding forgotten, 98
    key, 54
    locator, 234
Safety, 149–64
    and check-in systems, 156–58
    checklist, 163–64
    and con-artists, 158–61
    and distance caregiving, 149–60
    and elder abuse, 158
    home plan, 151–53

    and medications, 62–63
    precaution list, 153–55
    resources, 161–62
Sale/leaseback agreement, 94
Savings accounts, 54, 203
    and death, 200
    finding, 201
Savings bonds, 233
Savings certificates, 233
Schools
    records, 245
    as resources, 21, 145
Second opinion, 68, 184, 188
Securities and Exchange Commission, 91, 97
Self-defense, 161
Self-health care, 172
Senator, 112
Senior Centers, 12–13, 22, 170
Senior citizen discounts, 61, 90, 170
Senior escort programs, 158
Shared housing, 137, 144
Shopping, 156, 168, 169, 170
Skilled nursing facilities, 138
Sleep habits, 175
Smell problems, 175
Smoke alarms, 89
Smoking, 174
Social activities, 175
Social day care, 40, 73
Social Security, 93, 99, 236
    number, 56
    and paid care providers, 37–38
Social service organization, 11, 12, 40
Social worker, 107, 112
Speech/Language therapist, 178
Split-interest purchase, 96
Spouse
    and hospitalization, 71
    and Medicaid policies, 97, 125
State agencies
    department on aging, 20, 21, 38
    environmental protection department, 162
    health services department, 39
    Insurance Commission, 127

long-term care ombudsman, 38, 162
mental health department, 46, 189
public health department, 46, 189
secretary of state, 112
social services department, 39, 93, 94
tax office, 93
treasurer's office, 98
unemployment and workmen's
    compensation, 37–38
Stockbrokers, 91, 97
Stock certificate locator, 233
Storage, 201, 243
Stress, 44
Suicidal behavior, 213
Supplemental Security Income (SSI), 93
Support groups, 8, 45, 224
Surgery, 68, 177, 188

Task list, 33, 49
Tax(es), 66, 84, 119
    adviser, 88, 94, 97
    attorney, 91
    and estate planning, 105
    and hospitalization, 71
    and medications, 61
    postponement, 93
    relief, 12
    returns, 202, 237
Taxi, 169, 170
Teachers' associations, 21
Telecommunication for the deaf (TDD), 74, 112,
    161
Telephone bills, 78, 79, 88, 90, 97
Telephone calls
    for deaf and blind, 74
    and death notification, 198
    delegating, 69
    and fraud, 150, 159–60
    and hospitalization, 69–70
    reassurance services, 14, 157
    and staying connected, 223
    and taking notes, 10
Telephone directories, 24
    and caregiver help, 46–47

and community programs, 40
of elder's community, 11–12, 19
and emergencies, 54, 75
how to use, 11–12, 21
Telephone numbers
    emergency, 5, 54
    financial, 102
    which and where to keep, 50–51
Terminal illness, 196, 204
Testamentary trust, 105
Transportation, 165–71
    alternatives, 168–69
    checklist, 171
    and decision to stop driving, 165–68
    resources, 10, 12, 14, 170
    questions for getting help, 10
Travel
    costs, 79, 81, 90
    resources, 224
    safety, 155
    services for elderly, 210–11
Trust, 105, 235

Unions, 21
Urinary incontinence, 173
Urologist, 177
Utility bills, 97

Valuables, 70, 71, 240, 247
Veterans, 21, 93, 98, 128, 202
Vial of Life Program, 157
Videos, 21, 222–23
Vision problems, 97, 112, 175
Visiting nurse, 73
Visiting Nurses Association, 20, 40, 46, 48, 146,
    162, 196
Vital statistics, 199
Voice mail, 54
Volunteers, 12, 41, 73
    getting relief from, 45, 50
    opportunities for elders, 212

Wealth center, 99
Will, 104–6, 201–2, 23

If you are interested in having Joy Loverde speak at your company, church, club, school, business association, health-care facility, community center, or special event, please contact Silvercare Productions, 1111 N. Dearborn, Chicago, IL 60610, or call (312) 642-3611.